Certified Ophthalmic Technician
Exam Review Manual
Second Edition

Janice K. Ledford, COMT

EyeWrite Productions

Franklin, North Carolina

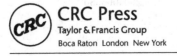

CRC Press
Taylor & Francis Group
Boca Raton   London   New York

CRC Press is an imprint of the
Taylor & Francis Group, an **informa** business

First published 2004 by SLACK Incorporated

Published 2024 by CRC Press
2385 NW Executive Center Drive, Suite 320, Boca Raton FL 33431

and by CRC Press
4 Park Square, Milton Park, Abingdon, Oxon, OX14 4RN

CRC Press is an imprint of Taylor & Francis Group, LLC

Ledford, Janice K.
    Certified ophthalmic technician exam review manual / Janice K. Ledford.-- 2nd ed.
        p. ; cm.
    Includes bibliographical references.
    ISBN 1-55642-648-8 (alk. paper)
    1. Ophthalmic assistants--Examinations, questions, etc. 2. Ophthalmology--Examinations, questions, etc.
    [DNLM: 1. Ophthalmology--Examination Questions. 2. Ophthalmic Assistants--Examination Questions.
    WW 18.2 L473ca 2004] I. Title.
    RE72.5.L427 2004
    617.7'0076--dc22

                                        2004000350

ISBN: 9781556426483 (pbk)
ISBN: 9781003522966 (ebk)

DOI: 10.1201/9781003522966

Dedication, First Edition

This book is dedicated to Cindy Bellamy, COT, and Ruth Bahr, COMT.

I was privileged to work alongside Cindy, if only for a short time. I have never seen anyone want to be a COT® as much as she did. She worked hard, and she deserves the status. Few people are as dedicated to or excited about our line of work as she is.

Ruth also rates a great deal of credit. Without her patient assistance, *Certified Ophthalmic Assistant Exam Review Manual* and *Certified Ophthalmic Technician Exam Review Manual* never would have been written. Her work at the Joint Commission on Allied Health Personnel in Ophthalmology® is evidence that she constantly is giving to the profession of ophthalmic medical assisting at every level.

Dedication, Second Edition

For the best eye buddies of 2003-4: Moya, Kate, Jin, and Charlie (better known as Dr. Kirby).

Contents

Acknowledgments, First Edition

Once again, I am indebted to some wonderful folks whose assistance allows me to do my favorite thing: write! Without Ruth Bahr, COMT (JCAHPO®), Bob Campbell, MD, and Jeff Freund, COMT, this book never would have been written. Ruth patiently endured all my queries related to exam criteria, and Jeff reviewed hundreds and hundreds of questions. My biggest thanks goes to Bob, my long-suffering editor, whose encouragement made it possible to finish a book that seemed to grow into overwhelming (and exhausting) proportions. I also appreciate the photographic assistance of Val Sanders, COT, CRA, of Eyesight Associates of Middle Georgia. Ginny Hansen, CO, COMT, Todd Hostetter, COMT, and Russell P. Edwards, MD, also helped by virtue of their expert advice.

Several questions were taken from *In-Office Training Manual and Series Review* from SLACK's Ophthalmic Technical Skills Series. Those question writers include: Norma Garber, COMT, Sheila Coyne Nemeth, COMT, Carolyn A. Shea, COMT, Ginny Hansen CO, COMT, Phyllis Rakow, COMT, NCLC, Michelle Herrin, COMT, and Budd Appleton, MD. Joe Hoffman's *Pocket Glossary of Ophthalmologic Terminology* (SLACK Incorporated) was used for many definitions.

Finally, I must thank my family. If it weren't for the three wonderful men I live with, I would never be able to write a single word. To Jim (who cooks, encourages, and never complains), T.J. (who keeps his knives and lighters away from my computer), and Collin (who thinks books are great...but, then, so are explosions): words can never express my appreciation for the three of you. And the four cats aren't bad, either!

Acknowledgments, Second Edition

My "family" at SLACK has changed over the years, but the company's dedication to serving the medical community is ever the same. My thanks to Amy McShane, John Bond, and Lauren Biddle Plummer.

For kind permission to use artwork and photos, I thank Norma Garber, Phyllis Rakow, Neil Choplin, and Russell Edwards. For answering questions as the work was in progress, my appreciation goes to Barbara Castleman (author, *The Low Vision Handbook*), Debbie Mason (JCAHPO®), Dr. Russell Edwards (co-author, *Visual Fields*), Dr. Johnny Gayton (co-author, *Refractive Surgery for Eyecare Paraprofessionals*), Dr. Charles Kirby, and Dr. Louis Schlesinger.

My "regular" family is growing, although there are fewer at home now. My husband Jim is a constant...patiently enduring this weird profession that has selected me. Collin (now a college student) is nearly on his own, but is still here to field my computer troubles. Gentlemen, I thank and love you both.

About the Author

Jan Ledford's first contact with the eyecare field occurred when she was about 7 years old. (We'll admit that this took place before eye exams were mandatory for school children, but don't tell Jan that we told you!) Her parents took her to an optometrist because her dad was very nearsighted. Sure enough, so was Jan. She remembers two things about that incident. First, the eye doctor was very nice because he had a great bag of goodies; if you were good, you could pick out several toys to take home. Second, once Jan got her glasses, she discovered that the trees had leaves and that the neighbors had a TV antenna on their roof.

About 2 years later, Jan got her first taste of the writer's life. She decided to write a book (at age 10!) about a talking hamster. When Mrs. Clark, her teacher, found out about the book, she had Jan read each chapter to the class. After Jan finished, the class applauded. That's all it took to make her love writing.

After entering the world of ophthalmic assisting in 1982, Jan advanced through the ranks until she earned her certification as an ophthalmic medical technologist. She brought with her not only a personal conviction about the importance of good vision, but an overwhelming desire to write. As of the printing of this second edition, she has 12 published books in the eyecare field.

Jan lives in Franklin, North Carolina, with her husband Jim, their youngest son (Collin, a college student and music major), and four cats (Munchkin, Boonie Rat, Angel, and Josey Dee). As a freelance medical writer and editor, she runs her own business called EyeWrite Productions. In addition to writing eyecare related material, she has branched into novels and short stories. You can check out her latest novel at www.millenniatech.info.

Introduction

Congratulations on becoming a certified ophthalmic assistant. I'm proud of you! Of course I hope that my book, *Certified Ophthalmic Assistant Exam Review Manual*, played a role in your success. So here you are, back for round two. Hopefully you've had a month or two to catch your breath, and now you're ready to go.

If this is your first experience with an exam review book, welcome! The modest cash investment you've made in purchasing this text will probably be repaid many times over with peace of mind and confidence. Peace of mind will come in knowing that there are questions covering every single exam content area listed in the most current exam criteria booklet. Confidence will be gained because first, you'll discover that you know more than you think you do. Second, because you'll identify any weak areas and bring them up to par before your exam.

If you use this book and follow through, it will help prepare you for the exam. It doesn't matter if you are in a formal training program or studying on your own, this book is for you!

If you used *Certified Ophthalmic Assistant Exam Review Manual*, you'll recognize the first chapter on studying for and taking exams. Whether you're reading it for the first time or skimming through it to refresh your study habits, you'll find useful information to help you "get ready to get ready." In *Certified Ophthalmic Technician Exam Review Manual, Second Edition*, I have added a section on taking the computerized practical exam to prepare you for what follows the written exam.

If it has been a few years since you took the ophthalmic assistant exam, you may want to use *Certified Ophthalmic Assistant Exam Review Manual* as a refresher course to review the background material. Then move right along into *Certified Ophthalmic Technician Exam Review Manual* as you prepare for your test.

My only wish is that we all lived close enough so we could celebrate together when you become a Certified Ophthalmic Technician!

This book also is useful for supervisors, teachers, physician-employers, office managers, and any others who need to assess the knowledge base of ophthalmic technician level personnel.

Note: The questions in this book were not taken from JCAHPO® files or previous tests. We have done our best to be sure that the information presented herein is accurate and up to date. The exam content areas, however, change from time to time. This book is not a product of JCAHPO®, who you should contact for current exam information. At some places, the content of this book might not follow the exact same order as the JCAHPO® criteria lists, but as of publication date all content areas were covered.

Brand Name Drug List

The following trademarked, brand name drugs appear in this book. Inclusion or exclusion of any drug does not imply endorsement (or lack thereof) of any drug or manufacturer by this author or the publisher.

Trade Name	Manufacturer
Acular	Allergan, Inc, Irvine, CA
AK-Beta	Akorn, Inc, Abita Springs, LA
AK-Sulf	Akorn, Inc, Abita Springs, LA
AK-Trol	Akorn, Inc, Abita Springs, LA
Alphagan	Allergan, Inc, Irvine, CA
Azopt	Alcon Laboratories, Fort Worth, TX
Betagan	Allergan, Inc, Irvine, CA
Betoptic	Alcon Laboratories, Fort Worth, TX
Betoptic-S	Alcon Laboratories, Fort Worth, TX
Bleph 10	Allergan, Inc, Irvine, CA
Blephamide	Allergan, Inc, Irvine, CA
Botox	Allergan, Inc, Irvine, CA
Celluvisc	Allergan, Inc, Irvine, CA
Chloroptic	Allergan, Inc, Irvine, CA
Ciloxan	Alcon Laboratories, Fort Worth, TX
Cortisporin	Monarch Pharmaceuticals, Bristol, TN
Cosopt	Merck & Co, Inc, West Point, PA
Daranide	Merck & Co, Inc, West Point, PA
Decadron	Merck & Co, Inc, West Point, PA
Diamox	Wyeth Pharmaceuticals, Philadelphia, PA
E-Pilo	CIBA Vision, Duluth, GA (discontinued)
FML	Allergan, Inc, Irvine, CA
Garamycin	Schering Corporation, Kenilworth, NJ
Genoptic	Allergan, Inc, Irvine, CA
GlaucTabs	Akorn, Inc, Abita Springs, LA
Gonak	Akorn, Inc, Abita Springs, LA
Goniosol	CIBA Vision, Duluth, GA
Healon	Pharmacia & Upjohn, Peapack, NJ
Humorsol	Merck & Co, Inc, West Point, PA
Hypotears	CIBA Vision, Duluth, GA
Icaps	Alcon Laboratories, Fort Worth, TX
Ilotycin	Dista Products/Eli Lilly and Company, Indianapolis, IN
Inderal	Wyeth-Ayerst Laboratories, Philadelphia, PA
Inflamase	Iolab, Claremont, CA
Iopidine	Alcon Laboratories, Fort Worth, TX
Ismotic	Alcon Laboratories, Fort Worth, TX
Lacri-Lube	Allergan, Inc, Irvine, CA
Lacrisert	Merck & Co, Inc, West Point, PA

Livostin	CIBA Vision, Duluth, GA
Lopressor	Novartis Pharmaceuticals, East Hanover, NJ
Lumigan	Allergan, Inc, Irvine, CA
Maxitrol	Alcon Laboratories, Fort Worth, TX
Monistat	Ortho Dermatological, Skillman, NJ
Murine	Ross Products Division, Columbus, Ohio
Muro 128	Bausch & Lomb, Inc, Tampa, FL
MZM	CIBA Vision, Duluth, GA
Naphcon A	Alcon Laboratories, Fort Worth, TX
Natacyn	Alcon Laboratories, Fort Worth, TX
Neosporin	Monarch Pharmaceuticals, Bristol, TN
Neo-Synephrine	Sanofi Pharmaceuticals, New York, NY
Neptazane	Wyeth Pharmaceuticals, Philadelphia, PA
Ocucaps	Akorn, Inc, Abita Springs, LA
Ocufen	Allergan, Inc, Irvine, CA
Ocuflox	Allergan, Inc, Irvine, CA
Ocupress	Otsuka America Pharmaceutical, Rockville, MD
Ocusert	Akorn, Inc, Abita Springs, LA
Ocuvite	Bausch & Lomb, Inc, Tampa, FL
Optipranolol	Bausch & Lomb, Inc, Tampa, FL
Oratrol	Alcon Laboratories, Fort Worth, TX
Osmitrol	Baxter Healthcare Corp, Deerfield, IL
Osmoglyn	Alcon Laboratories, Fort Worth, TX
Patanol	Alcon Laboratories, Fort Worth, TX
Pilocar	CIBA Vision, Duluth, GA
Pilopine	Alcon Laboratories, Fort Worth, TX
Plaquenil	Sanofi Pharmaceuticals, New York, NY
Poly-Pred	Allergan, Inc, Irvine, CA
Polysporin	Monarch Pharmaceuticals, Bristol, TN
Pred Forte	Allergan, Inc, Irvine, CA
Propine	Allergan, Inc, Irvine, CA
Quixin	Santen Inc., Napa, CA
Refresh	Allergan, Inc, Irvine, CA
Rescula	CIBA Vision, Duluth, GA
Tenormin	Zeneca Pharmaceuticals, Wilmington, DE
Tensilon	ICN Pharmaceuticals, Costa Mesa, CA
Timoptic	Merck & Co, Inc, West Point, PA
Timoptic XE	Merck & Co, Inc, West Point, PA
TobraDex	Alcon Laboratories, Fort Worth, TX
Tobrex	Alcon Laboratories, Fort Worth, TX
Toprol	Astrazeneca LP, Wilmington, DE
Travatan	Alcon Laboratories, Fort Worth, TX
Trusopt	Merck & Co, Inc, West Point, PA
Valium	Roche Products, Humaco, Puerto Rico
Vasocon-A	CIBA Vision, Duluth, GA
Vasosulf	CIBA Vision, Duluth, GA

Vira-A   Monarch Pharmaceuticals, Bristol, TN
Viroptic   Monarch Pharmaceuticals, Bristol, TN
Viscoat   Alcon Laboratories, Fort Worth, TX
Voltaren   CIBA Vision, Duluth, GA
Xalatan   Pharmacia & Upjohn Co, Bridgewater, NJ
Zovirax   Glaxo Wellcome, Research Triangle Park, NJ

Chapter 1

Study and Test Taking Strategies

Setting goals seems to be a human passion. Perhaps it wasn't too long ago when you set your sights on becoming certified as an ophthalmic assistant. Now you have chosen a new goal, expanding your horizons and increasing your value to your employer and patients. Your decision also means that you must once again buckle down and study. Allow the worthiness of your major goal (becoming certified) to empower and motivate you as you take the smaller steps that move you in that direction, whether it is breaking brand new technical ground or just completing the day's reading. Having a goal when studying will give you purpose and motivation to continue and to improve.

Hitting the Books

Reading

It may be your tendency to zip through everything you read. In and of itself, fast reading is not necessarily poor reading. The key in study-reading is to comprehend what you read, regardless of your reading speed.

Here are several suggestions to help you increase your reading speed and comprehension:

1. Before you start, know why you are reading. In our case, we are seeking to learn and understand new material. We are looking for information.
2. Glance over the headings and subheadings to get a quick grasp of the main ideas before you start to read. (More on this later.)
3. When reading the material for the first time, take it slow and easy.
4. Look up any words you don't know. Increasing your vocabulary will increase your cumulative reading speed.

There are several bad habits that will slow down your reading. You'll need to eliminate them. Here are the biggest offenders:

1. Using your finger or a pencil to track along as you read. Stop!
2. Moving your whole head as you read across the page. Instead, you should move your eyes across the page, keeping your head still.
3. Moving your lips as you read. (To find out if you do this, hold a pencil between your lips while reading. Don't bite or grip it with your teeth, just hold it gently between your lips. If the pencil waggles and falls out as you read, you're afflicted.) The remedy is to put the pencil between your lips every time you read for a week or so. Concentrate on holding the pencil still. You eventually should be able to retrain yourself and kick the habit.
4. Reading each and every word independently. Train yourself to read groups of words instead.

Here are a few pointers on careful reading:

1. Before you start, have an idea of what you're looking for. Skim the headings to see what's in store.
2. As you read, concentrate. Pay attention to what you're doing. (More on this later when we talk about studying.)
3. Relax. Try to leave your problems behind. Focus on your reading.
4. Don't panic if you didn't seem to catch on after reading the material for the first time. Don't freeze up. Read it again.
5. Take a break after 45 minutes or so of straight reading. Reward your brain and body with a nice long stretch. Your eyes need a break, too. But instead of closing them, gaze at something far off in the distance for a minute or so. This will relax the ciliary muscle and help prevent accommodative spasms.

Good reading habits can be learned. With practice (and you'll be getting plenty of that) your reading skills gradually will improve. If you have a serious reading deficit, you should consider professional counseling.

Study Strategy

Like reading, good study habits can be learned and developed over time. If you have an interest in the topic, it's easier to study. Your study will be focused and purposeful. In the exam/certification game, your study habits can make or break you.

With a little bit of preplanning, your study time will become second nature. To avoid hit-and-miss studying, you need to plan your work and then work your plan, as the saying goes.

First, choose a place where you will study. I know you've heard this before, but here it is again: study in the same place every session. The ideal study conditions include:

1. Ample desk room—a good writing surface with enough space to spread out. If you can create a place for yourself that is off-limits to anyone else, that would be best. Then you can leave your materials there and won't have to regather everything each session.
2. Good lighting.
3. Comfortable temperature. It'll be hard to study huddled over a space heater in the basement!
4. A sturdy, comfortable chair (but not too comfortable).
5. No distractions, or at least minimal distractions. We usually think of distractions as noise. But there may be visual distractions as well. It's even been suggested that you remove your family's picture from your desk. Certainly studying in front of a window would be distracting. We'll talk about minimizing family interruptions later.

There is one other type of distraction, and it is the toughest one to eliminate: drifting brain syndrome. These are internal distractions—thoughts that pop into your head unbidden as you try to study. You may be worried about paying the rent, or your daughter's football game (she's the quarterback!). The dog may have fleas and the 2-year-old may have temper tantrums. But try to put these things aside (as much as possible) when it comes to your study time. All of your problems will still be there when you've finished your assignment.

Once you've carved out your study niche, the next item on the agenda is *when* you are going to study. You need to be a good time manager since you probably are adding studying to an already crowded schedule of obligations. Trying to fit your studying between or after other activities can lead to problems.

To help decide what time is best for you, consider what part of the day you are at your best. Try to schedule at least some of your studying during that time. For "morning people" that means studying early in the a.m., before the day really starts. If mornings make you queasy, study at night after the kids are in bed. Either the early morning or late night time-slot will eliminate or at least minimize those family distractions we were looking at earlier.

So set a definite time you will study and commit yourself to it. Set your highest priorities and put them on your calendar. For now, studying for your exam will have to be one of those high priorities. Add other less important things around your study schedule as you are able. To help carve out your study time, try to become more efficient in your other tasks. Check out books that will teach you how to save time doing things. Your family won't cave in if you don't squeeze your own orange juice or fix your own car. This need to study is temporary, anyway. Teach the kids how to make their own peanut butter and pickle sandwiches. (And ask them to make you one, too, while they're at it!)

How long should you study each day? That depends in part on how much time you have before the date of your exam. But you should understand that the shorter the study time, the sooner you will forget what you've learned. In fact, you may not learn much at all, having stored the information in your short-term memory. Most of it will pop back out after the test. As you plan your study time, remember that to be efficient and avoid fatigue you should give yourself about a 10-minute break after each 45 minutes or so of intense study. This break time must be included as a vital part of your study schedule.

Having a schedule for study has several advantages:

1. It puts you in control. You're never biting your pencil wondering what to do next.
2. It decreases anxiety. You're not overwhelmed by all those areas in the criteria book because you know that each item is going to be covered.

3. You'll work efficiently. You'll know you have a certain number of pages to cover. You won't spend time flipping through your book trying to decide what to read next.

Organizing a Study Schedule

Creating a study schedule for yourself is a matter of listing what you need to accomplish, then fitting that into the amount of time you have. Giving yourself 6 months to get ready for the exam should be plenty of time to proceed at a relaxed but steady pace. Of course everyone is different, and each person's situation is different. Here is a sample 6-month plan. You'll need to accomplish the work listed regardless of the time you have available, so this should be helpful whether you have 6 months or (heaven forbid!) 6 weeks.

Month 1—Obtain criteria booklet and application. Review requirements and obtain necessary paperwork (proof of home study course, CPR card, etc.). Assemble study texts, use index and table of contents to find information appropriate to content areas. Make a list of the topics and corresponding page numbers. Don't waste time with material that's not on the test. Decide when you will study (days and times) and divide the material accordingly. Allow several weeks before the test for review.

Month 2—Send in application. (This way you'll be ahead of schedule if there are any problems with your paperwork.) Begin working your study schedule.

Month 3—When you receive notification regarding your eligibility to take the exam, call and register (up to 3 months in advance). Continue following your study schedule.

Month 4—Continue study plan.

Month 5—Finish study plan. Register for exam if you haven't already done so. Make arrangements for travel and accommodations if necessary.

Month 6—Review. Eat properly and get plenty of rest. Final days of review.

Square What?

Okay. So you've chosen a time and a place. You've formulated a study schedule, which gives you a goal for each study period. Your textbook is on your desk and you're ready to get to work. What's next?

Next is a nifty little method of study-reading called the SQ3R method.[1] The letters and number are a mnemonic for the five general steps for good study-reading. SQ3R stands for survey, question, read, recite, and review. Here's how you use it:

1. Survey. Before reading, leaf through the pages you will be covering that study period. Skim the headings and subheadings, pictures, and captions for an overview. As you glance over the material, you will probably recognize some of it. This scanning process will give direction to your reading and aid in your concentration.

2. Question. From your survey, formulate some mental questions about what you're going to read. What do you expect to learn? Turn the headings into questions. For example, suppose you notice the sub-heading "Control Centers for Eye Movements." You could ask yourself: "What are these control centers? How do they affect eye movements? What types of eye movements are there?" Also ask yourself, "What do I already know about this topic?" These questions will help you concentrate as you look for the answers. If you have trouble doing this, you may want to write down your questions for several sessions just to get the hang of it. After that you can just keep them in your head.

3. The 3 R's.

   a. The first R refers to the actual reading. As you read, you will be checking for three items. First, you'll be looking for the answers to the questions you've just formulated during the questions stage. Second, you'll be paying attention to those "little extras"—captions, graphs, illustrations, and so forth. Third, you'll be alert to words and phrases that are boldface, italicized, or underlined. Look up any words you don't know.

   b. The second R stands for recite. After you have read a short portion of your assignment, stop and summarize it. Condense the material into key words and phrases that will jog your brain to remember what you just read. There are several ways to do this. First, recite orally. This gives you extra stimulation by involving your hearing, not just your vision. A second method of recitation is to go back over the material quickly and underline or mark important parts of the text. Underline only key words or phrases, not entire sections. This gives you something to refer back to when you begin to review for the test. Later, when you glance over the material and see the words you highlighted, you will remember what you read about. A third way to recite is to make notes after you read, jotting down key words and main ideas. Summarize the material in your own words. You could even make these notes on index cards, creating valuable flash cards for later study.

  c. The last R of SQ3R stands for review. After you've read the entire assignment, stopping several times to recite, you should go back over all the material one more time. Look over the headings again, thinking over what each section was about. Let the marked words and phrases jog your memory.

Each day when you sit down to study, it's important to crank up and get going; don't dawdle or daydream. Remember to take a break every hour or so, and be sure to reward yourself in some way when you've finished. Watch TV or take a bubble bath. (But be cautious about rewarding yourself with food! If you do that, you'll probably find that you have gained a bit of weight by exam time. Then the self-discipline you've been using to study will have to be applied to dieting. Yuck! So if you want to reward yourself with a snack, stick to fruit and carrot sticks. You'll be doing yourself a favor!)

How to Prepare for a Test

Managing Pretest Stress[2]

Things might have been pretty relaxed when all you had to do was read. Now that test time is close, the heat is on and you may be feeling the pressure. Actually, a moderate amount of stress is good for you. Not enough stress and you will be too carefree. Too much stress and you will freeze. So let's take an honest look at the situation.

What's at stake? This is not a do-or-die risk we're talking about. You can retake the test if you need to. Regardless of the results, you will come out alive.

Uncontrolled stress is not productive. Focused stress can help you think more clearly and sharpen your perception. Later we'll talk about what to do if you panic during the test. But for now you need to relax so you can review productively. There are several ways you can prepare yourself for the exam and control your stress.

  1. Academic preparation. Study! The other three are useless without this one. We'll talk about reviewing in a minute. If you've taken the test before, use the printout of missed items to strengthen weak areas.

  2. Psychological preparation. Be positive! Build yourself up. Remind yourself of the benefits of passing. I was studying for my COMT® exam in 1988 during the Summer Olympics. I got a lot of encouragement in watching the competition. I knew I never would compete in an Olympics, but I had my own important job to do. I was reaching for my own gold. The athletes didn't give up, no matter what; I wouldn't either. By the same token, don't compare yourself with others. Look at the test as an opportunity rather than an adversary. Avoid self-pity by planning to reward yourself in some way when the test is over.

It might seem odd to mention this as part of your psychological readiness, but avoid smoking or chewing gum when you study. You won't be allowed to do either during the exam, and that might throw you off.

Get some information about the test itself. Knowing what to expect reduces stress. How many questions are there? What topics are covered? What type of questions might be asked? How long do you have to take the test? Do you need to take pencils and paper? All these are answered for you in the criteria booklet. Talk to friends who have taken the test. If possible, visit the test site ahead of time. Then the place will be familiar.

If you have a history of panic during tests, consider getting counseling ahead of time. Also, there are some things you can do to handle panic—we'll cover them later.

3. Physical preparation. The proper food and rest are important all the time, not just the night before the test. In the weeks before the exam, reduce sugars and increase protein and vitamins.

4. Logistical preparation. Make early plans for getting to the test site, and have a backup plan ready. Be sure to take your admission card and ID. Don't forget your watch and any materials you may require.

Computer-itis

All of the JCAHPO® exams are now computerized, but even if you've never put your hand to a mouse (or aren't sure what a mouse is!), don't let it stop you. The friendly folk at your testing center will be glad to help. (In fact, the first thing they'll do when you report to take your exam is give you a tutorial in navigating the computer and test.) Here are a few key computer terms to help you out:

- Monitor—the television-like view screen. You won't have to mess with this; the testing center will do any necessary turning on or adjusting.
- Keyboard—the typewriter-like component that you use to enter answers and make selections.
- Mouse—a palm-sized device with one to three buttons on it that can also be used to enter answers and make selections. Moving the mouse (rolling it around on the pad) moves the cursor; clicking a button on the mouse enters a choice.
- Cursor—a tiny line, rectangle, or arrow on the monitor that shows you "where you are"; it's like a pointer. Its position can be manipulated by the mouse or keyboard.

If you don't have a computer at home or office, use one at your local library. Libraries often have brief classes of a couple hours to introduce patrons to the computer. Have a librarian help you access and move around on the JCAHPO® website (www.jcahpo.org). And relax a little. The computer allows you to mark a question and come back to it later, as well as change an answer. No more worrying whether or not you filled in the circle completely, or got off on your numbering. Hooray! Plus, you get an immediate pass/fail notice, although it's not official until you hear from JCAHPO®.

Review Techniques

Study Material

Now that your reading is completed, you are armed with some formidable study aids. From the "question" part of SQ3R you have study questions. From the "recite" portion of SQ3R you have a highlighted text, written notes, and flash cards. Dig out your old home study course test. (Make sure the answers are correct!) Some books have questions at the end of the chapter. Of course you will plan on spending time daily with *this* book. Ask questions at work about anything you don't understand. Talk to others who have taken the test, picking their brains for what they remember. You might want to make a new schedule to allot specific review times for specific material.

The test includes diagrams (you match the letter on the picture to the correct answer), and single best answer questions (a statement or questions followed by four possible answers, one of which is best, ie, multiple choice). Both of these types of questions call for recognition more than recall. If your study methods include asking yourself the tougher type of fill-in-the-blank and short answer questions, you will be even better prepared for the actual exam.

Another study aid you might consider is a formal ophthalmic technician review class. These are offered by various individuals and groups across the country, often over a weekend. There are many advantages to such a course. First, you get the benefit of being taught by someone who has already taken and passed the exam. Second, you have a chance to rub shoulders with others who, like you, are determined to pass. Finally, you'll come home with handouts and other valuable material to study. The class also should help you identify your areas of strength and weakness. Instead of a review course, you might attend a seminar or similar meeting that allows you to choose the courses you want. Select classes that fall into the six content areas. Contact JCAHPO® for a list of review classes and seminars near you.

The Review Session

Successful review starts long before a mere 4 weeks before your exam. It's a fact of life: you have to study the material before you can review it! But since you made and followed a reading schedule months ago, you're ready to review. Way to go!

When reviewing, start with the material you feel least confident about, then move to the easier topics. Don't worry yourself over what they "might" ask. Concentrate on what they're *most likely* to ask.

Go back through your reading material, skimming what you marked. The next time you go through it, skip over what you know. Then grab a friend and recite, going over the material verbally. If you didn't make flash cards when you originally read the material, do so now. This will help you with memorization (covered in the next section).

How to Memorize[3]

1. Repetition—practice! This is another reason why flash cards are so great. You can pull them out of your pocket while you are in the line at the grocery store and get in 5 minutes of study. Going over the material again and again really gets it into your conscious and subconscious brain.

2. Association—associate new information with something you already know. Mnemonics are merely intended to assist the memory. Do you remember Roy G. Biv? That silly name is the mnemonic used to memorize the colors in the spectrum. Each letter of the name stands for one of the hues. (Can't remember them? Go look it up!) You can make up mnemonics for yourself. Here's one of my favorites: the edges of a minus lens bow inward, giving the lens the appearance of being *caved* in. That's how I remember that it is a con*cave* lens.

3. Stimulation—of as many senses as possible. Making your own note and flash cards serves several purposes. Your sight is stimulated by reading, touch by writing, and hearing when you recite aloud.

Fifteen to 20 minutes at a time of intense memorization is enough. Committing material to memory is more intense than reading, so give yourself more frequent breaks.

Study Groups

Study groups can be a great way to review the material for your exam. Besides having someone to study with, group study can help you manage stress simply by knowing that you are not alone. There are others who are going through the rigors of test preparation! If you met once a week for 7 weeks, you could cover one content area at each session and have a final session for review. Ideally, find someone who has already taken and passed the exam to function as group leader. If there is no one available to be your guide, you could take turns at being the facilitator. One person might be especially good at a particular task or subject, and could conduct that review.

Use the same strategies in a group as you have for your own private study. Set a specific time and place, and be sure to schedule breaks. This is a review, so everyone should have a good understanding of the material already. Try to stay on target, but don't forget that laughter is a great stress-reliever. Listen and learn from each other. Someone else may have a fresh perspective that will "turn the lights on" some topic you may have been struggling with. Or they may have a mnemonic or some other way of remembering that will help you. Be sure to share your discoveries, too. Use the same review materials in the group as you would alone. Another idea is to ask each group member to write several multiple choice questions to share. Perhaps each person could do a different content area.

Remember SQ3R? Use R2 (recite) as a study aid. Have a partner scan your reading material and ask you to:

1. Explain the chapter title, headings, and subheadings
2. Define bold or italicized words and phrases
3. Answer questions based on the pictures and tables
4. Answer questions from the end of the chapter, this book, or old home-study tests.

There are several cautions about study groups, however. If someone in the group tends to panic or be anxious, he or she can affect the whole group. If encouragement doesn't help, you might have to ask him or her to refrain from making negative comments. If you are beginning to get upset yourself, it might be better to study alone.

Close Encounters of the Examination Kind

Test Day

Actually, let's look at test day minus one. The day before your exam needs to be as laid-back as possible. Eat well and get plenty of rest. Plan what you will wear tomorrow (something comfortable!) so you won't be scrambling around in the morning. If you must travel to the test site and spend the night before, allow plenty of time to get there. If possible, drive by the test center so you know where it is. Ideally, go in and look at the room itself. This will help you psychologically. Review your notes for about an hour before going to bed. Refuse to upset yourself by thinking about all that you don't know.

Now the alarm rings, and it's test day. Get up early enough so you're not rushed. Eat a good breakfast that includes protein, but avoid eating anything too heavy in the 2 hours just prior to test time. Remember your admission card, ID, watch, any materials. Arrive early. If possible, choose a distraction-free seat. It's probably best not to talk to others about the test beforehand. Try to relax. Focus on being calm and self-confident.

How to Take a Test

Listen to the proctor. Read instructions carefully. Be sure to enter your name and number correctly.

If you are not taking the test on a computer, the exam is machine scored. Fill in the circle completely. If you want to change an answer, be sure to erase it thoroughly. A question with two responses is automatically marked wrong. Use the right type of pencil (usually those supplied).

Before you start, find out how many questions there are. When your time is half up, if you haven't worked to the halfway point, go there anyway.

In the COT® exam, there are 3.5 hours to answer about 210 questions. That is 1 minute per question. Use this information to pace yourself.

Read the entire question before looking at the answers. Think of an answer before you read the choices. Read each choice before marking an answer.

A multiple choice question is actually a group of true/false questions. Try out each answer. Does it make the statement true or false? One answer will be "truer" than all the rest. Answer the easy questions, then go back to those you're not sure of or have to figure out. You might jot a note or two about a tougher question to help you when you come back. When you've been through the test once and are going back to answer the harder questions, continue to pace yourself. If you feel the need for spending a while on a question, move on again and come back later. Your subconscious will be looking through your brain files for the answer while you move on. When you come back to a question, it may have "soaked" long enough and the answer will come right to you. Multiple choice questions often contain one answer that is obviously wrong, one or two answers that appear reasonable, and one or two correct answers. (If there are two, one is more correct than the other). If the answer to a question is not obvious to you, eliminate any answers that you are sure are wrong. Then try to pick the best answer from those that are left.

If the question involves math, read the problem carefully. What do they want to know (lens power, cylinder axis, minus cylinder)? Estimate the answer before you start the actual calculations.

Every now and then one question will contain the answer or hints to another. Lucky you! But don't waste too much time looking back through trying to find something.

Do your best to concentrate on one question at a time.

Beware of the following words: none, most, never, always, must, only, all, some, usually, sometimes, every, many, few, often, seldom, more, equal, less, best, good, bad, worst, exactly, and may. If used in the question, be sure to read very carefully.

If you finish before time is up, go back over the test to those questions you weren't sure about.

Managing Panic

If you panic, stop (before you freeze). Take a brief break. Close your eyes. Talk to yourself. Remember all you did to prepare for the exam. Then breathe! Inhale for 3 seconds, hold it for 12, then exhale for 6 seconds. This helps even out your blood gas level and puts you in control. Remind yourself that you know what to do—you have a plan. Refocus on the task at hand. Concentrate on one question at a time, not on the whole test. Imagine yourself in a familiar setting, at work on a task that you know you can perform. Hold that thought, then get back to work.

Taking the Practical Exam

Once you receive the good news that you've passed the written test, you realize that not only have you accomplished something great, but you get to take another test! Certification as an ophthalmic technician requires that you also pass a practical exam. As of 2003, the practical is given in the form of a computer simulation.

After you pass the written COT® exam, JCAHPO® will issue an application for the skill evaluation. After the application is approved, you will be issued a CD-ROM tutorial. JCAHPO's® website also has an abbreviated form of the tutorial. The skill evaluation covers retinoscopy and refinement (ie, refractometry), keratometry, lensometry (NON-automated), applanation tonometry, phoria/tropia testing, and automated visual fields. At publication, the retinoscopy/refinement and lensometry sections are in plus cylinder; minus cylinder will be available soon. You have 1.5 hours to complete the exam.

References

1. Carman RA, Adams WR. *Study Skills: A Student's Guide for Survival*. New York, NY: John Wiley & Sons; 1972.
2. Elifson JM, Gordon B. *Strategies for Passing the Georgia Regents' Exam*. Raleigh, NC: Contemporary Publishing Co of Raleigh, Inc; 1982.
3. Lass A, Wilson E. *The College Student's Handbook*. New York, NY: David White; 1965.

Bibliography

Berry M. *Help Is on the Way For: Tests*. Chicago, IL: Childrens' Press; 1985.
Lenz E, Shaevitz MH. *So You Want to Go Back to School*. New York, NY: McGraw-Hill; 1977.

Chapter 2

Clinical Optics

1. **The range of wavelengths in the visible spectrum is:**
   a) 100 to 400 nanometers
   b) 400 to 800 nanometers
   c) 450 to 650 nanometers
   d) 400 to 800 meters (m)

2. **Immediately on either side of the visible spectrum are the invisible light segments of:**
   a) Infrared and ultraviolet
   b) X-rays and radio waves
   c) Gamma rays and laser
   d) Microwaves and radar

3. **Which color has the longest wavelength?**
   a) Red
   b) Yellow
   c) Green
   d) Blue

4. **Geometric optics includes:**
   a) The origin of light waves and particles
   b) The effects of media on the path of light
   c) How light travels through the eye
   d) Physics of the visible light spectrum

5. **When light bounces back from an object, this is known as:**
   a) Reflection
   b) Refraction
   c) Transmission
   d) Index of refraction

6. **In reflection, the light rays that hit the object or interface between media with different indices of refraction are called:**
   a) Incident rays
   b) Reflected rays
   c) Refracted rays
   d) Transmitted rays

7. **In optics, a *medium* (or *media*, plural) is:**
   a) An object that refracts light
   b) An object that emits light
   c) An object that reflects light
   d) An object through which light passes

8. **When light passes through a transparent medium, it may travel straight through (transmission) or its path may be altered. This altering or bending property of a medium is known as:**
   a) Reflection
   b) Refraction
   c) Absorption
   d) Tropism

9. **The ray of light that enters a transparent medium is termed:**
   a) Incident ray
   b) Divergent ray
   c) Emergent ray
   d) Parallel ray

10. **If light passes through a lens and the rays are spread *apart* on exiting, this is known as:**
    a) Index of refraction (IR)
    b) Convergence
    c) Zero vergence
    d) Divergence

11. **If light passes through a lens and the rays are bent *toward* each other on exiting, this is known as:**
    a) IR
    b) Convergence
    c) Zero vergence
    d) Divergence

12. **A comparison of the speed of light in air to the speed of light through a substance is:**
    a) IR (Snell's Law)
    b) Angle of refraction
    c) Internal reflection
    d) Optical interference

13. **The denser the substance, the more slowly light passes through it, and:**
    a) The lower the IR
    b) The higher the IR
    c) The more transparent it is
    d) The more suitable it is for use as an ophthalmic lens

14. **The IR of crown glass is:**
    a) 0
    b) 1.00
    c) 1.33
    d) 1.50

15. **Light traveling through a prism will be bent toward the prism's:**
    a) Apex
    b) Base
    c) Center
    d) Smallest angle

16. **The image of an object viewed through a prism:**
    a) Is real and shifted toward the base
    b) Is virtual and shifted toward the base
    c) Is real and shifted toward the apex
    d) Is virtual and shifted toward the apex

17. **A 1.00 diopter prism bends light:**
    a) 1 centimeter (cm) at a distance of 1 cm from the prism
    b) 1 m at a distance of 1 cm from the prism
    c) 1 cm at a distance of 1 m from the prism
    d) 1 m at a distance of 1 m from the prism

18. **A 2.00 diopter prism displaces an object 1 cm at a distance of:**
    a) 0.2 m
    b) 0.5 m
    c) 1.5 m
    d) 5.0 cm

19. **The displacement of an object 5 cm at a distance of 1 m would require prism of:**
    a) 0.5 diopters
    b) 1.0 diopters
    c) 2.0 diopters
    d) 5.0 diopters

20. **At a distance of 2 m, a 12 diopter prism would displace an object:**
    a) 6 cm
    b) 2.4 m
    c) 24 cm
    d) 6 m

21. **A spherical lens refracts light:**
    a) Not at all
    b) In one direction only
    c) Equally in every direction
    d) At 90 degrees from its axis

22. **A 1.00 diopter spherical lens focuses light at:**
    a) 1/2 m
    b) 1 m
    c) 1 cm
    d) 1 yard (yd)

23. **The point at which a lens forms an image (whether real or virtual) is the:**
    a) Nodal point
    b) Conoid of Sturm
    c) Focal length
    d) Focal point

24. **All of the following regarding the optical center of a lens is true *except*:**
    a) It always coincides with the geometric center of the lens
    b) Light rays passing through it are not refracted
    c) It also is known as the nodal point
    d) It should be centered in line with the patient's visual axis

25. **The focal length of a lens:**
    a) Is the distance between the lens and the focal point
    b) Is the dioptric power of the lens
    c) Is the point where light is focused
    d) Is related to the axis of the cylinder

26. **Because the focal point of a minus lens is virtual, the focal length of a minus lens:**
    a) Cannot be calculated
    b) Is likewise virtual
    c) By contrast, is real
    d) Is insignificant

27. **Which of the following is the formula for finding focal length?**
    a) IR = speed of light in air/speed of light in substance
    b) P = C/D
    c) P = 1/F
    d) U + P = V

28. **What is the focal length of a 5 diopter lens?**
    a) 5 m
    b) 0.5 m
    c) 2 m
    d) 0.2 m

29. **A lens has a focal length of 33 cm. What is its dioptric power?**
    a) 0.03 diopters
    b) 0.3 diopters
    c) 3 diopters
    d) 30 diopters

30. **Designate each lens characteristic as belonging to: a) Plus spherical lenses, or b) Minus spherical lenses.**
    A. Virtual image
    B. Converges light
    C. Used to correct presbyopia in the emmetrope
    D. Minifies
    E. Barrel distortion
    F. Concave
    G. Thicker in the middle
    H. Used to correct aphakia
    I. Magnifies
    J. Used to correct myopia
    K. Two prisms placed base to base
    L. Diverges light
    M. Pincushion distortion
    N. Used to correct hyperopia
    O. Convex
    P. Two prisms placed apex to apex
    Q. Thinner in the middle
    R. Real image

31. **All of the following regarding cylindrical lenses are true *except*:**
    a) They are used to correct astigmatism
    b) They have power in one axis, but no power in the axis 90 degrees away
    c) They focus light in a line
    d) They are plus power lenses

32. **The direction of the line of light as focused by a plus power cylindrical lens:**
    a) Is virtual and cannot be placed
    b) Is 90 degrees from the axis
    c) Is aligned with the axis
    d) Is 45 degrees from the axis

33. **Light passing through a cylindrical lens is focused in two lines perpendicular to each other and separated by an area known as:**
    a) Induced interval
    b) Sturm's interval
    c) Anterior focal interval
    d) Posterior focal interval

34. **The light rays in the above-mentioned interval are projected in the shape of a:**
    a) Circle
    b) Prism
    c) Curve
    d) Cone

35. **Within the Conoid of Sturm, the area where the image would be most clearly focused is:**
    a) The circle of least confusion
    b) The cone of least confusion
    c) The focus of least confusion
    d) The secondary focal point

36. **An optical cross is a means of:**
    a) Marking the optical center of a lens
    b) Calculating the amount of induced prism
    c) Determining whether or not a lens is polarized
    d) Indicating the dioptric power of a lens

37. **What is the prescription of the lens represented by the following optical cross (Figure 2-1)?**
    a) +3.00 sphere
    b) +3.00 + 3.00 X 090
    c) +3.00 + 3.00 X 180
    d) +3.00 + 6.00 X 090

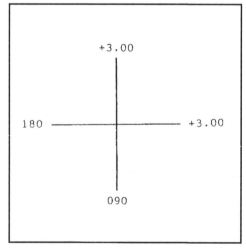

Figure 2-1.

38. What is the prescription of the lens represented by the following optical cross (Figure 2-2)?
    a) Plano - 2.25 X 180
    b) - 2.25 - 2.25 X 180
    c) Plano + 2.25 X 090
    d) Plano - 2.25 X 090

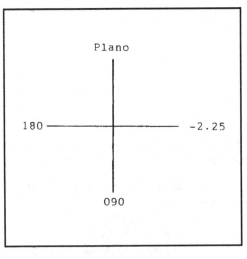

Figure 2-2.

39. What is the prescription of the lens represented by the following optical cross (Figure 2-3)?
    a) -1.25 + 2.00 X 135
    b) + 2.00 - 1.25 X 135
    c) + 2.00 - 3.25 X 045
    d) -3.25 + 2.00 X 045

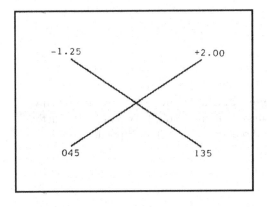

Figure 2-3.

40. The ocular media consist of:
    a) The lens correction for ametropia
    b) Contact lenses and intraocular lenses
    c) The eyelid, sclera, uvea, and optic nerve
    d) The tear film, cornea, humors, and lens

41. **Which of the following ocular structures has the *highest* refractive power?**
    a) Tear film
    b) Cornea
    c) Lens
    d) Aqueous and vitreous (combined)

42. **The primary goal of the eye's components is to:**
    a) Interpret what is seen
    b) Focus incoming light onto the lens
    c) Focus incoming light onto the retina
    d) Maintain proper intraocular pressure

43. **Images pass through the optic nerve and thence to the:**
    a) Lateral geniculate body, chiasm, occipital cortex, and brain stem
    b) Optic tract, lateral geniculate body, and cerebral cortex
    c) Chiasm, optic tract, lateral geniculate body, and occipital cortex
    d) Chiasm, optic tract, lateral geniculate body, and cerebellum

44. **Which situation is depicted by the following progression of figures (Figures 2-4 through 2-6)?**
    a) Correction of simple myopic astigmatism with minus sphere and plus cylinder
    b) Correction of simple hyperopic astigmatism with minus sphere and plus cylinder
    c) Correction of simple myopic astigmatism with plus sphere and minus cylinder
    d) Correction of compound myopic astigmatism with minus sphere and plus cylinder

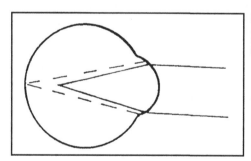

Figure 2-4. Drawing by Holly Hess. Reprinted with permission from Ledford J. *Exercises in Refractometry*. Thorofare, NJ: SLACK Incorporated; 1990.

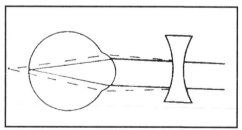

Figure 2-5. Drawing by Holly Hess. Reprinted with permission from Ledford J. *Exercises in Refractometry*. Thorofare, NJ: SLACK Incorporated; 1990.

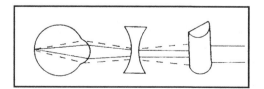

Figure 2-6. Drawing by Holly Hess. Reprinted with permission from Ledford J. *Exercises in Refractometry*. Thorofare, NJ: SLACK Incorporated; 1990.

45. Which situation is depicted by the following progression of figures (Figures 2-7 and 2-8)?

a) Correction of myopia with minus sphere

b) Correction of simple myopic astigmatism with minus sphere

c) Correction of simple myopic astigmatism with minus cylinder

d) Correction of myopia with minus cylinder

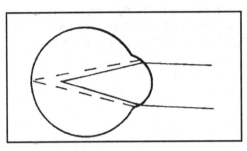

Figure 2-7. Drawing by Holly Hess. Reprinted with permission from Ledford J. *Exercises in Refractometry*. Thorofare, NJ: SLACK Incorporated; 1990.

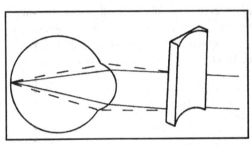

Figure 2-8. Drawing by Holly Hess. Reprinted with permission from Ledford J. *Exercises in Refractometry*. Thorofare, NJ: SLACK Incorporated; 1990.

46. Which situation is depicted by the following progression of figures (Figures 2-9 through 2-11)?

a) Correction of simple myopic astigmatism with minus sphere and plus cylinder

b) Correction of mixed astigmatism with minus sphere and plus cylinder

c) Correction of compound myopic astigmatism with minus sphere and plus cylinder

d) Correction of compound myopic astigmatism with plus sphere and minus cylinder

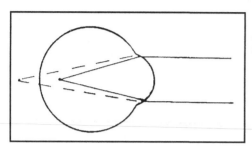

Figure 2-9. Drawing by Holly Hess. Reprinted with permission from Ledford J. *Exercises in Refractometry*. Thorofare, NJ: SLACK Incorporated; 1990.

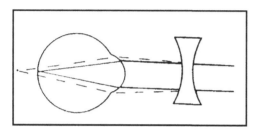

Figure 2-10. Drawing by Holly Hess. Reprinted with permission from Ledford J. *Exercises in Refractometry*. Thorofare, NJ: SLACK Incorporated; 1990.

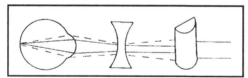

Figure 2-11. Drawing by Holly Hess. Reprinted with permission from Ledford J. *Exercises in Refractometry*. Thorofare, NJ: SLACK Incorporated; 1990.

47. **Which situation is depicted by the following progression of figures (Figures 2-12 through 2-14)?**
    a) Correction of simple hyperopic astigmatism with plus sphere and plus cylinder
    b) Correction of compound hyperopic astigmatism with plus sphere
    c) Correction of compound hyperopic astigmatism with plus sphere and plus cylinder
    d) Correction of compound hyperopic astigmatism with plus sphere and minus cylinder

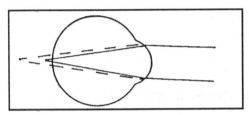

Figure 2-12. Drawing by Holly Hess. Reprinted with permission from Ledford J. *Exercises in Refractometry.* Thorofare, NJ: SLACK Incorporated; 1990.

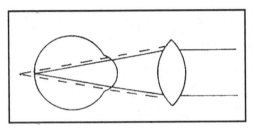

Figure 2-13. Drawing by Holly Hess. Reprinted with permission from Ledford J. *Exercises in Refractometry.* Thorofare, NJ: SLACK Incorporated; 1990.

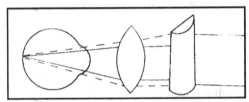

Figure 2-14. Drawing by Holly Hess. Reprinted with permission from Ledford J. *Exercises in Refractometry.* Thorofare, NJ: SLACK Incorporated; 1990.

48. **All of the following are true regarding the accommodative reflex *except*:**
    a) It is stimulated by a blurred image
    b) It is not a true reflex
    c) It is required for viewing distant objects
    d) It includes convergence, miosis, and focusing

49. **When the ciliary muscle relaxes:**
    a) Close objects become clear
    b) There is more focusing power
    c) The lens is pulled thinner
    d) The zonules go limp

50. **The main reason one's accommodative ability decreases with age is due to:**
    a) One's arms becoming shorter
    b) Laxity of the ciliary muscle
    c) Laxity of the zonules
    d) Hardening of the crystalline lens

51. With accommodation fully relaxed, what is the patient's point of clearest vision?
a) The far point
b) The near point
c) Accommodative amplitude
d) Range of accommodation

52. The "power" of a myopic eye itself is:
a) Minus
b) Plus
c) Neutral
d) Irrelevant

53. The retinoscope provides information on the patient's refractive status by:
a) Reflecting light off the patient's cornea
b) Reflecting light off the patient's retina
c) Reflecting light off the patient's lens
d) Projecting light from the examiner's retina

54. The streak retinoscope permits:
a) No comparison of principal meridians
b) Neutralization of individual ocular meridians
c) Subjective measurement of nonverbal patients
d) Correction of plus cylinder only

55. All of the following are components of the streak retinoscope *except*:
a) Light and power sources
b) Condensing lens and mirror
c) Rotating lens system
d) Focusing sleeve

56. Raising or lowering the focusing sleeve of a streak retinoscope:
a) Rotates the streak to evaluate all meridians
b) Changes the vergence of the light leaving the instrument
c) Permits measuring of hyperopia or myopia
d) Adjusts for the examiner's own refractive error

57. The plane mirror effect is used in streak retinoscopy because:
a) It is easier to use the instrument with the sleeve up
b) It is easier to use the instrument with the sleeve down
c) This projects parallel light rays into the eye
d) This projects converging light rays into the eye

58. If a streak retinoscope is habitually placed flat on the table:
a) This is an acceptable practice
b) The lenses may get scratched, causing a distorted reflex
c) The mirror will be jarred out of alignment
d) The filament may bend, causing a distorted streak

59. A working lens is required in retinoscopy in order to:
a) Simulate working at infinity
b) Simulate working at 10 m
c) Simulate working at 66 cm
d) Simulate working at 14 inches (in)

60. **Standard retinoscopy working distance is:**
    a) 50 cm
    b) 66 cm
    c) 75 cm
    d) 88 cm

61. **If you use a retinoscopy working distance that is closer than the standard, your working lens will need to be:**
    a) The same at any working distance
    b) More plus power than standard
    c) More minus power than standard
    d) One should work at the standard distance only

62. **Which of the following can be determined with the most accuracy using a streak retinoscope?**
    a) Sphere power
    b) Sphere axis
    c) Cylinder power
    d) Cylinder axis

63. **The magnitude of a refractive error can often be evaluated by noting all of these streak qualities *except*:**
    a) Brightness
    b) Width
    c) Speed
    d) Height

64. **In streak retinoscopy, the *intercept* is:**
    a) That part of the streak that is reflected from the pupil
    b) When the streak is swept at 90 degrees
    c) When the streak is swept at 180 degrees
    d) The part of the streak that falls on the patient's iris

65. **If you sweep the retinoscope streak across the patient's pupil and the reflex travels in the same direction as the intercept, this is known as:**
    a) Neutrality
    b) "With" motion
    c) "Against" motion
    d) Luminosity

66. **Most retinoscopists prefer to neutralize "with" motion because:**
    a) They work in plus sphere
    b) They work in minus sphere
    c) "Against" motion can be difficult to evaluate
    d) "With" motion can be difficult to evaluate

67. **One can convert any situation to "with" motion by adding:**
    a) Plus cylinder
    b) Minus cylinder
    c) Enough plus sphere
    d) Enough minus sphere

68. **One matches the retinoscope streak to the axis of the refractive error by:**
    a) Rotating the sleeve until there is an unbroken line
    b) Raising the sleeve until there is an unbroken line
    c) Lowering the sleeve until there is an unbroken line
    d) Turning the instrument until there is an unbroken line

69. **As the measurement approaches neutrality, the reflex will become:**
    a) Dimmer, slower, and longer
    b) Brighter, wider, and faster
    c) Brighter, narrower, and faster
    d) Brighter, wider, and slower

70. **At the point of neutrality, the reflex will:**
    a) Be clearer to the patient
    b) Appear as a fine line
    c) Seem to blink on and off
    d) Disappear entirely

71. **All of the following regarding use of the streak retinoscope are true *except*:**
    a) Keep the room lights low
    b) Keep both of your eyes open
    c) Measure the patient's right eye with your right eye
    d) When using your right eye, hold the retinoscope in your left hand

72. **To help stabilize the retinoscope and maintain alignment:**
    a) Rest it against your brow or spectacle frame
    b) Rest the handle against your cheek
    c) Rest your elbow on the exam chair arm rest
    d) Rest it against the phoropter

73. **If your patient is *not* dilated for retinoscopy, instruct him to look at:**
    a) Your nose
    b) The retinoscope light
    c) A target on the near card
    d) A target on the distance chart

74. **If your patient is fully dilated for retinoscopy, you should:**
    a) Evaluate the full reflex
    b) Concentrate on the peripheral portion of the reflex
    c) Concentrate on the central portion of the reflex
    d) Instill dilation reversal drops until the pupil is 3 mm

75. **In streak retinoscopy, if the streak is vertical, you should:**
    a) Sweep the streak up and down
    b) Sweep the streak left to right
    c) Sweep the streak in a circle
    d) Turn the streak to the horizontal

76. **In your initial retinoscopy evaluation (using the proper working lens), you note that the patient has "against" motion in every meridian. This indicates:**
    a) Myopia
    b) Hyperopia
    c) Mixed astigmatism
    d) Compound hyperopic astigmatism

77. In your initial retinoscopy evaluation (using the proper working lens), you note that the patient has "with" motion in one meridian and "against" motion in the other. This indicates:
    a) Simple hyperopic astigmatism
    b) Mixed astigmatism
    c) Compound hyperopic astigmatism
    d) Compound myopic astigmatism

78. In your initial retinoscopy evaluation (using the proper working lens), you note that the patient seems to be neutralized already. You should:
    a) Record your measurement as Plano sphere
    b) Double check for a high refractive error
    c) Retinoscope through the cross cylinder
    d) Remove the working lens and check again

79. You are working in plus cylinder using a working lens. You see "with" motion at 090 degrees and neutralize this with +1.50 sphere. You now see "with" motion at 180 degrees. Next you should:
    a) Set the cylinder axis at 180 and add cylinder until the reflex is neutralized
    b) Set the cylinder axis at 090 and add cylinder until the reflex is neutralized
    c) Neutralize the horizontal meridian with sphere, then the vertical meridian with cylinder
    d) Convert the "with" motion at 180 degrees to "against", and neutralize with sphere

80. You are working in minus cylinder using a working lens. You have neutralized "with" motion at 045 degrees. You turn to 135 degrees and now see "with" motion. You should:
    a) Give cylinder at 135 degrees until the reflex is neutral
    b) Give cylinder at 45 degrees until the reflex is neutral
    c) Neutralize at 135 degrees by giving more plus sphere, then neutralize at 45 degrees with cylinder
    d) Neutralize at 135 degrees by removing sphere, then neutralize at 45 degrees with cylinder

81. If not using the built-in retinoscopy lens on the refractor, when the measurement is complete you must:
    a) Record the refractor setting in the patient's chart
    b) Add 1.50 sphere for the working distance
    c) Subtract 1.50 sphere for the working distance
    d) Fog the patient and re-evaluate the reflex

82. Which of the following patients would probably be the easiest to retinoscope?
    a) A patient who has had a corneal graft
    b) A patient with a posterior subcapsular cataract
    c) A patient with an intraocular lens (IOL) implant
    d) A patient who has had refractive surgery

83. All of the following are true regarding fogging *except*:
    a) It may be used during cross cylinder testing
    b) It may be used to help prevent giving too much minus
    c) It can be used as an alternative to occlusion
    d) It can be used to relax accommodation

84. Fogging is accomplished by:
    a) Placing a polarized lens in front of the eye to blur the vision
    b) Placing the Bagolini lens in front of the eye to blur the vision
    c) Placing enough plus power in front of the eye to blur the vision
    d) Placing a Maddox rod in front of the eye to blur the vision

85. **The astigmatic dial is useful for:**
    a) Finding the exact cylinder power
    b) Refining astigmatic correction
    c) Finding the exact cylinder direction
    d) Estimating the cylinder axis

86. **The astigmatic dial looks like:**
    a) A telephone dial
    b) A clock face
    c) A circular grid
    d) A circle with horizontal lines

87. **When using plus cylinder, if the patient says that all the lines on the astigmatic dial seem to be equally clear:**
    a) The test is over; proceed directly to cross cylinder refinement
    b) Turn the cylinder axis knob 45 degrees and ask again if any lines are darker
    c) Add +0.50 sphere and ask again if any lines are darker
    d) Open the aperture and try the test with both eyes together

88. **In plus cylinder, if the patient says that the lines on the astigmatic dial running from 12 to 6 are clearer, you will set your axis cylinder at:**
    a) 090 degrees
    b) 180 degrees
    c) 0 degrees
    d) 045 degrees

89. **In minus cylinder, if the patient says that the lines on the astigmatic dial running from 12 to 6 are clearer, you will set your axis cylinder at:**
    a) 045 degrees
    b) 090 degrees
    c) 135 degrees
    d) 180 degrees

90. **When using the astigmatic dial, once you have set your axis, you should:**
    a) Add cylinder until all lines are equally clear
    b) Add sphere until all lines are equally clear
    c) Use the cross cylinder until all lines are equally clear
    d) Remove the dial and refine with the cross cylinder

91. **The cross cylinder is used:**
    a) To refine cylinder axis and power
    b) To refine sphere axis and power
    c) To refine sphere and cylinder power
    d) To refine sphere and cylinder axis

92. **Before cross cylinder testing, it is important to:**
    a) Be close to the sphere power endpoint
    b) Refine sphere power to the endpoint
    c) Measure for bifocal add
    d) Balance the two eyes

93. **On cross cylinder testing:**
    a) The power of the sphere should always be measured first, then its axis
    b) The axis of the sphere should be measured first, then its power
    c) The power of the cylinder should be measured first, then its axis
    d) The axis of the cylinder should always be measured first, then its power

94. **When refining the axis using minus cylinder, you should follow which dot on the cross cylinder?**
    a) Red
    b) White
    c) Blue
    d) There are no dots on the cross cylinder

95. **You are using plus cylinder, and are refining cylinder power. The present cylinder power is +0.50. The patient says that the letters are more clear when the white dot is showing on the cross cylinder. What should you do now?**
    a) Rotate the axis toward the white dot
    b) Change the cylinder power to zero
    c) Change the cylinder power to +1.00
    d) Stop because you are at the end point

96. **You are using minus cylinder, and are refining cylinder power. The present cylinder power is -1.00. The patient says that the letters are more clear when the white dot is showing on the cross cylinder. What should you do now?**
    a) Switch to plus cylinder
    b) Change the cylinder power to -1.50
    c) Change the cylinder power to -0.50
    d) Change the sphere power by +0.50

97. **The generally accepted end point for the cross cylinder test (for either axis or power refinement) is:**
    a) When the first choice is better than the second choice
    b) When the second choice is better than the first choice
    c) When the two choices appear equal
    d) When the patient states her vision is most comfortable

98. **Duochrome technique of refining sphere depends on:**
    a) The fact that green rays are refracted more than red rays
    b) Red rays will appear orange, and green rays will appear blue
    c) The patient having normal color vision
    d) Contrast sensitivity to red light as opposed to green light

99. **The duochrome test is useful to:**
    a) Determine a patient's color vision
    b) Help prevent giving too much plus
    c) Help prevent giving too much minus
    d) Refine cylinder correction

100. **Before beginning the duochrome test, do all of the following *except*:**
    a) Occlude one eye
    b) Get an accurate distance correction
    c) Place a red filter in front of the eye
    d) Fog with +0.50 sphere

101. If the patient says that the letters in the red panel are sharper, you should:
   a) Record this as your end point
   b) Add more cylinder
   c) Add more plus power to the sphere
   d) Add more minus power to the sphere

102. The end point for the duochrome test generally is accepted to be when the letters:
   a) In the red panel are clearer
   b) In the green panel are clearer
   c) Are equally clear in both panels
   d) In both panels no longer are visible

103. If a patient is red-green color blind:
   a) The duochrome test cannot be used
   b) Place a Maddox rod in front of the right eye
   c) Place a Bagolini lens in front of the right eye
   d) Refer to left and right sides instead of red and green

104. If the patient is accommodating during retinoscopy or refractometry, this may result in:
   a) A prescription that has over-plus
   b) A prescription that has over-minus
   c) A prescription without necessary cylinder correction
   d) A prescription that will cause the eyes to relax too much

105. All of the following may be used to reduce or eliminate accommodation *except*:
   a) Duochrome test
   b) Bringing the distant eye chart closer
   c) Fogging
   d) Topical cycloplegics

106. A patient whose prescription is inaccurate due to accommodation will have to:
   a) Relax accommodation in order to see clearly when wearing the correction
   b) Have prism in the lenses to reduce diplopia
   c) Accommodate in order to see clearly when wearing the correction
   d) Have a bifocal for near vision

107. If a patient is known to be myopic:
   a) One need not worry about accommodation
   b) One must still reduce or eliminate accommodation
   c) The eye has no ability to accommodate
   d) Avoiding too much minus is not critical

108. The ideal distant refractometric measurement:
   a) Leaves vision slightly blurred on the plus side to avoid over-minusing
   b) Is slightly over-minused in order to stimulate accommodation
   c) Causes as much accommodation as possible
   d) Gives the clearest vision possible and relaxes accommodation

109. Which of the following will give the refractometrist the most useful information regarding the patient's refractive status?
   a) The history
   b) The muscle balance check
   c) The slit lamp exam
   d) The fundus exam

110. **All of the following patients could have alterations to their refractive status *except*:**
    a) A diabetic
    b) A pregnant woman
    c) A patient with cataracts
    d) A patient taking allergy shots

111. **In order to avoid contaminating the distant measurement, refractometry should be performed prior to:**
    a) Tonometry
    b) Dilation
    c) Pupil exam
    d) Muscle balance testing

112. **A slit lamp exam is useful before refractometry in order to:**
    a) Determine if astigmatism is present
    b) Measure the intraocular pressure (IOP)
    c) Check the clarity of the media
    d) Determine if refractometry is needed

113. **Which of the following is *true* regarding the difference between "refraction" and "refractometry"?**
    a) Objective measurement is used in refractometry
    b) Only refractions are written in the patient's chart
    c) Clinical judgment is used in a refraction
    d) Only a licensed practitioner can perform refractometry

114. **Before beginning the refractometric measurement on an adult, it is important to:**
    a) Explain the procedure
    b) Have an auto-refractor reading
    c) Make sure she can read 20/20
    d) Instill artificial tears to clear the tear film

115. **Using a trial frame might be preferable over using the refractor (phoropter) when:**
    a) The patient has facial deformities
    b) The patient already wears glasses
    c) Performing retinoscopy first
    d) The patient has a head tremor

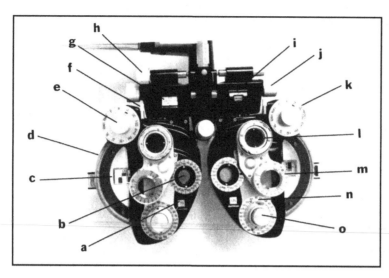

Figure 2-15. Photo by Jim Ledford, PA-C, PhD. Reprinted with permission from Ledford J. *Exercises in Refractometry.* Thorofare, NJ: SLACK Incorporated; 1990.

116. **Label the parts of the refractor (Figure 2-15).**

Pupillary distance (PD) adjusting knob	Sphere power
Cylinder power	3 diopter sphere dial
Cylinder power dial	Level
Prism	Aperture
PD scale	Cylinder axis dial
Sphere dial	Aperture knob
Aperture convergence lever	Leveling screw
Cross cylinder	

117. **All of the following are appropriate adjustments to the refractor (phoropter) before starting the distance measurement** *except*:
   a) Set to the patient's PD
   b) Set to an appropriate vertex distance
   c) Converge the apertures
   d) Make sure the instrument is level

118. **In general, the first step in refractometry is to:**
   a) Correct as much of the refractive error as possible with cylinder
   b) Correct as much of the refractive error as possible with sphere
   c) Find the cylinder power using the cross cylinder
   d) Find the cylinder axis using the cross cylinder

119. **When offering the patient changes in spheres, a good general rule is to:**
   a) Refine the axis before the power
   b) Offer more plus first
   c) Offer more minus first
   d) Always use minus cylinder

120. **You have no prior record on your young patient, and he has never worn glasses. His vision is 20/80 uncorrected. A correction of -1.50 sphere brings his vision up to 20/30. -2.00 and -2.50 sphere gives no improvement in vision. Your next step should be:**
    a) Record the final measurement as -1.50 sphere
    b) See if -1.75 or -2.25 sphere will help
    c) Use the duochrome test
    d) Check for astigmatism

121. **You are measuring a patient from scratch (no retinoscopy, lensometry, prior records, etc.). Your best spherical correction is +2.00 sphere for 20/60 vision. You use the astigmatic dial and find that the lines are equally black with cylinder -1.50 X 180. What is your next step?**
    a) Change the sphere setting to +2.75
    b) Change the sphere setting to +1.25
    c) Refine the cylinder axis
    d) Record the measurement

122. **Your patient reads 20/20 with the following setting: -2.00 + 1.25 X 065. To refine the sphere, you first change the sphere setting to -1.75. The patient says the 20/20 line is now a bit blurred. You show her -2.00 again, and she says it is clearer. Now you change the sphere to -2.25. The patient says the letters are smaller but clearer. What is your next step?**
    a) See if -2.50 helps
    b) Record the final measurement as -2.25 + 1.25 X 065
    c) Record the final measurement as -2.00 + 1.25 X 065
    d) Record the final measurement as -1.75 + 1.25 X 065

123. **Your healthy patient has clear media, although you have not looked at the retina. Your best refractometric measurement yields only 20/40 vision. What should you do next?**
    a) Record the measurement as final
    b) Label that eye as amblyopic
    c) Get a pinhole vision
    d) Perform a stereo test

124. **If your patient has over 6.00 diopters of astigmatism:**
    a) You cannot use the refractor
    b) The cross cylinder will not work
    c) The fogging technique must be used
    d) An auxiliary cylinder lens must be used

125. **Balancing is performed:**
    a) With the right eye occluded
    b) With the left eye occluded
    c) With both eyes open
    d) While standing on one foot

126. **The purpose of balancing is:**
    a) To ensure that the vision is the same in each eye
    b) To make sure that the eyes are accommodating equally
    c) To ensure that the measurement in each eye is as nearly the same as possible
    d) To make sure that the eyes are not crossing

127. **To test for the reading add, the standard near card is placed:**
    a) At the distance preferred by the patient
    b) At 10 in
    c) At 14 in
    d) At 20 in

128. **The general rule for determining the reading add is to:**
    a) Give the least amount of plus possible
    b) Give the maximum amount of plus
    c) Go by the standard age chart
    d) Never give more than +3.00

129. **When measuring the refractive error of a patient with low vision, it is helpful to:**
    a) Speak a little more loudly and slowly
    b) Urge her to choose quickly between lens options
    c) Use larger steps (ie, 0.50 or larger) for refinement
    d) Use smaller steps of 0.25 to increase accuracy

130. **Each of the following procedures can affect the refractometric measurement *except*:**
    a) Pterygium removal
    b) Blepharoplasty
    c) Nasolacrimal probing
    d) Chalazion removal

131. **A patient with a cataract probably will show evidence of what type of refractive shift?**
    a) Increased myopia
    b) Decreased myopia
    c) Increased presbyopia
    d) Increased hyperopia

132. **All of the following can cause a hyperopic shift in the refractometric measurement *except*:**
    a) Orbital mass
    b) Macular swelling
    c) Elevated blood sugar
    d) Corneal edema

133. **The disease/condition that is most likely to cause refractometric shifts from one exam to the next is:**
    a) Diabetes
    b) Hypertension
    c) Hyperthyroid
    d) Gout

134. **The ocular disease/condition that is most likely to cause refractometric shifts from one year to the next is:**
    a) Astigmatism
    b) Keratoconus
    c) Contact lens over-wear
    d) Glaucoma

135. **The effective diameter (ED) of a lens is measured:**
    a) Vertically across the eyewire opening of the frame
    b) Horizontally across the eyewire opening of the frame
    c) Diagonally across the eyewire opening of the frame
    d) Across the center of the lens blank

136. **If an aphake is corrected with glasses, he might require +12.00. If he wears a contact lens, he might need +14.00. This increase in power with a decrease in distance to the cornea is a product of:**
    a) Axial length
    b) Vertex distance
    c) Pupillary distance
    d) Spherical equivalence

137. **Vertex distance is defined as:**
    a) The distance between the back of the glasses lens and the front of the eye
    b) The distance between optical centers
    c) The distance between the front and back of the spectacle lens
    d) The distance between the visual axis of the right and left eye

138. **Vertex distance becomes increasingly important:**
    a) The more compulsive the patient is
    b) The worse the patient's vision is
    c) The stronger the correction is
    d) The weaker the correction is

139. **Vertex distance should be included with the refractometric measurement if:**
    a) The patient's vision is 20/20
    b) The patient's vision is 20/40 or worse
    c) The correction is 4.00 diopters or more
    d) The correction is 4.00 diopters or less

140. **Vertex distance is measured with a(n):**
    a) Vertexometer
    b) Distometer
    c) Lensometer
    d) Ophthalmometer

141. **In order to convert the change of lens power required as one goes from the vertex distance of a trial frame to the vertex distance of the patient's spectacles, one must:**
    a) Use a conversion scale
    b) Read the numbers on the caliper
    c) Use the spherical equivalent
    d) Transpose to minus cylinder

142. **If the optician adjusts the lens to account for vertex distance:**
    a) The lens power may not match the original prescription
    b) The patient will complain of diplopia
    c) The vision will not be as good as in the patient's record
    d) There will be induced prism

143. **Prism is prescribed in order to:**
    a) Redirect the line of sight
    b) Improve vision
    c) Cure amblyopia
    d) Cure strabismus

144. **Prism options for prescription lenses include all of the following *except*:**
    a) Decentration
    b) Press-on
    c) Power compensation
    d) Ground-in

145. **Which patient might benefit the most from prism correction?**
    a) One with a horizontal imbalance of 1.50 diopters
    b) One with a vertical imbalance of 1.50 diopters
    c) One with -2.00 sphere OD and -1.00 sphere OS
    d) One with intermittent esotropia

146. **A press-on prism would be ideal for:**
    a) A patient gradually recovering from a palsy
    b) A patient with a 20 diopter esotropia
    c) A patient with a 15 diopter exotropia
    d) A patient with a permanent palsy

147. **Placing the optical centers closer to the patient's nose is termed:**
    a) Outward decentration
    b) Inward decentration
    c) Superior decentration
    d) Inferior decentration

148. **The patient is a myope. The optical center of the right lens is in line with the visual axis. The optical center of the left lens is 2 mm to the left. This induces a prismatic effect of:**
    a) Base in
    b) Base out
    c) Base up
    d) Base down

149. **A hyperopic 12-year-old bent his glasses while playing basketball. The optical center of the right lens is 1.5 mm too high and the left lens is 2.00 mm too low. This induces a prismatic effect of:**
    a) Base up right eye, base up left eye
    b) Base down right eye, base down left eye
    c) Base up right eye, base down left eye
    d) Base down right eye, base up left eye

150. **The patient requires 12 prism diopters base in, right eye. Instead of giving this all in one lens, the prescriber will probably give:**
    a) 6 diopters base in OD, 6 diopters base in OS
    b) 6 diopters base out OD, 6 diopters base out OS
    c) 6 diopters base in OD, 6 diopters base out OS
    d) 6 diopters base out OD, 6 diopters base in OS

151. **The patient requires 12 prism diopters base up, left eye. Instead of giving all this in one lens, the prescriber will probably order:**
    a) 6 diopters base up OD, 6 diopters base up OS
    b) 6 diopters base down OD, 6 diopters base down OS
    c) 6 diopters base up OD, 6 diopters base down OS
    d) 6 diopters base down OD, 6 diopters base up OS

152. **Prentice's rule for induced prism is found by:**
    a) Multiplying vertex distance by millimeters of decentration
    b) Multiplying millimeters of decentration by pupillary distance
    c) Dividing centimeters of decentration by lens power
    d) Multiplying centimeters of decentration by lens power

153. **A +4.25 sphere lens is decentered *in* by 0.50 cm. What is the prismatic effect?**
    a) 2.125 base in
    b) 2.125 base out
    c) 8.5 base in
    d) 8.5 base out

154. **The patient requires a -6.50 spherical correction and 3.00 prism diopters base up in the right eye. How much should the lens be decentered, and in which direction?**
    a) 2.16 mm below the optical axis
    b) 2.16 mm above the optical axis
    c) 4.6 mm below the optical axis
    d) 4.6 mm above the optical axis

155. **The patient is wearing +2.75 sphere OD and +2.00 sphere OS. The lenses are decentered in by 2.75 mm OD and 1.25 mm OS. What is the approximate total prismatic effect?**
    a) 1.0 prism diopters base in
    b) 0.50 prism diopters base out
    c) 10.0 prism diopters base in
    d) 0.1 prism diopters base out

156. **Which lens is *least* likely to cause its wearer grief if decentered horizontally?**
    a) +12.00 sphere
    b) -6.00 sphere
    c) +4.00 sphere
    d) -2.00 sphere

157. **Slab-off lenses are most useful in:**
    a) High myopia
    b) Presbyopia
    c) Anisometropia
    d) Ametropia

158. **Each of the following patients is anisometropic. Which one might benefit from a slab-off?**
    a) The one with diplopia when reading
    b) The one with diplopia at a distance
    c) The one with headaches in the morning
    d) The one with severe amblyopia

159. **When prescribing bicentric lenses, the patient should be told all of the following** *except***:**
    a) Slab-off lenses are more expensive
    b) There will be a faint line across the lens at the level of the bifocal
    c) The slab-off will help the eyes work together better
    d) The slab-off will improve the patient's near acuity

160. **The slab-off lens is fashioned by:**
    a) Decentering the near vision segments
    b) Grinding away a portion of the lower segment
    c) Decentering the distant vision segment
    d) Grinding away a portion of the upper segment

161. **Bicentric grinding works by:**
    a) Shifting the optical centers of the lower segments closer to one another
    b) Shifting the optical centers of the upper segments closer to one another
    c) Shifting the optical center of the lower segment closer to the optical center of the upper segment
    d) Shifting the optical center of the upper segment closer to the optical center of the lower segment

162. **Successful adaptation of the patient to aphakic (cataract) spectacle lenses includes:**
    a) Careful presurgical measurements
    b) Patient education for realistic expectations
    c) Implantation of a secondary IOL
    d) Discouraging the patient from using contact lenses

163. **High plus lenses have the disadvantage of disrupting depth perception and changing the position of the entire visual field. This is caused by:**
    a) Minification
    b) Magnification
    c) The concave lens shape
    d) "With" motion

164. **A cataract lens that is ground with a smaller optical portion and another carrier portion is called a:**
    a) Lenticular lens
    b) Full-field lens
    c) Kryptok lens
    d) Bicentric lens

165. **The advantage of the full-field aphakic lens is:**
    a) It is thinner
    b) Improved depth perception
    c) A wider field of view
    d) A full range of focal distances

166. **A disadvantage of the lenticular lens is:**
    a) It has a thicker center
    b) The reduction of spectacle-ring scotoma
    c) It cannot be made with plastic
    d) It is not cosmetically pleasing

167. **The advantages of aspheric lenses include all of the following** *except*:
    a) It is available in both lenticular and full-field form
    b) The PD and vertex distance are not as critical
    c) A thinner center
    d) A wider field of view

168. **All of the following are true regarding spectacle-ring scotoma** *except*:
    a) The thicker the lens, the more pronounced the scotoma becomes
    b) It causes a Jack-in-the-Box effect
    c) It is eliminated by using crown glass as a lens material
    d) It is caused by the prismatic effect of the lens edges

169. **In addition to the prescription itself, it is vital to include which of the following measurements for aphakic eyewear?**
    a) Front and back surface powers
    b) Base curve and refractive index
    c) Lens material and size limitations
    d) Vertex distance and PD

170. **Of those listed, the best lens available for aphakia is:**
    a) Combining the lenticular form with aspheric surfaces
    b) Combining the full-field form with bicentric grinding
    c) Plastic full-field
    d) Crown glass lenticular

171. **The two basic divisions of low vision aids are:**
    a) Optical and nonoptical
    b) Tactile and auditory
    c) Low and high magnification
    d) Magnifiers and telescopes

172. **Examples of optical low vision aids include:**
    a) Magnifiers, telescopes, and high-powered bifocals
    b) Reading glasses, large print, and yellow filter
    c) Stand magnifier, Braille, and high-intensity lamp
    d) Closed circuit television, and books on tape

173. **Examples of nonoptical low vision aids include:**
    a) High-powered reading glasses, and magnifying glass
    b) Writing guide, high illumination lighting, and large print
    c) Magnifiers, telescopes, and closed circuit television
    d) Magnifying page, Braille, and reading guide

174. **Patients with reduced visual fields would be expected to benefit most from:**
    a) Optical magnification
    b) Optical minification
    c) Increased illumination
    d) Infrared rejection lens

175. **Magnification functions as a low vision aid by:**
    a) Shortening the viewing distance
    b) Shortening the working distance
    c) Increasing the size of the retinal image
    d) Using only one lens

176. **The "X" system of manufacturing low vision aids:**
    a) Is based on a 10 cm working distance
    b) Is based on a 40 cm working distance
    c) Is based on a 1 m working distance
    d) Is not based on any particular working distance

177. **A magnifying glass with a power of 10 X has a dioptric power of:**
    a) 4
    b) 10
    c) 25
    d) 40

178. **The image in a magnifying lens is clear at 5 cm from the page. What is the magnifying power of the lens?**
    a) 2 X
    b) 5 X
    c) 8 X
    d) 20 X

179. **The patient has a 30 diopter hand magnifier. What distance should he hold it from the page to get the clearest magnified image?**
    a) 3.33 cm
    b) 4.50 cm
    c) 7.52 cm
    d) 75.00 cm

180. **Advantages of telescopes modified for near versus a regular magnifier include:**
    a) Increased working distance
    b) Comparative lightness and reduced size
    c) Relatively wide field
    d) All of the above

181. **An elderly person with hand tremors might do well with any of these low vision aids *except*:**
    a) A stand magnifier
    b) A hand magnifier
    c) A page magnifier
    d) A reading stand with light

182. **A college law student with low vision might benefit most from using:**
    a) A reading telescope
    b) A stand magnifier
    c) A hand magnifier
    d) A computerized low vision scanner (CCTV)

183. **A visual aid that was successful in the office but not at home most likely has failed because:**
    a) The power was not really adequate
    b) The lighting at home is not adequate
    c) The patient is using her eyes too much
    d) The patient is incapable of using the aid

Chapter 3

Basic Ocular Motility

Note: Directions of gaze are given from the viewpoint of the patient, *not the examiner. For example, "to the right" means the patient's right. When taking the certification exam, read the questions very carefully.*

1. **Adduction means the eye is turning:**
   a) Outward (toward the ear)
   b) Inward (toward the nose)
   c) Up
   d) Down

2. **If the eye is *depressed*, it is:**
   a) Turning in
   b) Closed
   c) Recessed into the orbit
   d) Turning down

3. **Which muscles have *only* a primary action?**
   a) MR and LR
   b) SR and IR
   c) SO and IO
   d) SR and SO

4. **Which muscles are elevators?**
   a) SR and IR
   b) SR and SO
   c) IO and SR
   d) IO and SO

5. **As a tertiary action, both oblique muscles:**
   a) Adduct
   b) Abduct
   c) Intort
   d) Elevate

6. **Which muscles are primarily torsional muscles?**
   a) IR and IO
   b) MR and LR
   c) IR and SR
   d) SO and IO

7. **Which muscles act to depress the eye?**
   a) IR and SO
   b) SR and IO
   c) IR and SR
   d) IO and SO

8. **Which muscles adduct the eye as a tertiary action?**
   a) SR and IR
   b) SO and IO
   c) SR and SO
   d) IR and IO

9. **Which is an example of yoked muscles?**
   a) RLR and LMR
   b) RLR and RMR
   c) RLR and LLR
   d) RIR and LIR

10. **Which muscles are synergists for horizontal movement with the MR?**
    a) IO and IR
    b) IR and LR
    c) SR and SO
    d) SR and IR

11. **Which muscles are antagonists for depression with the IR?**
    a) SR and SO
    b) SR and IO
    c) MR and LR
    d) SO and IO

12. **If one eye is obviously turned in, out, up, or down when you perform a simple external evaluation of the patient, this deviation is a(n):**
    a) Lazy eye
    b) Phoria
    c) Tropia
    d) Vergence

13. **A phoria is exhibited when:**
    a) The patient is malingering
    b) Fusion is disrupted
    c) The patient is fusing
    d) The patient has diplopia

14. **The difference between a phoria and an intermittent tropia is:**
    a) The patient experiences diplopia with the phoria but not with the intermittent tropia
    b) The phoria rarely is controlled and the intermittent tropia always is controlled
    c) The phoria usually is controlled and the intermittent tropia always is uncontrolled
    d) The phoria usually is controlled and the intermittent tropia sometimes is controlled

15. **An adult patient with a tropia has either:**
    a) Amblyopia or anisometropia
    b) Prism or slab-off lenses
    c) Diplopia or suppression
    d) Fusion or stereopsis

16. Label the following on Figure 3-1:
  Esotropia
  Exotropia
  Hypertropia
  Hypotropia
  Orthophoria

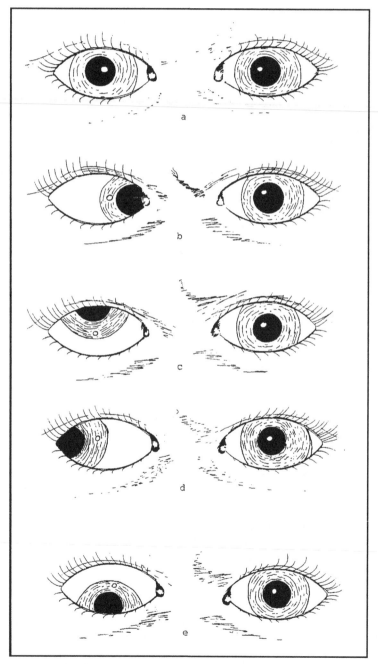

a

b

c

d

e

Figure 3-1. Drawing by Holly Hess. From *The Crystal Clear Guide to Sight for Life*. Starburst Publishers. Used by permission.

17. **An intermittent horizontal tropia might be aggravated by all of the following** *except*:
    a) Inattention
    b) Reading
    c) Illness
    d) Fatigue

18. **Your patient has an exodeviation that is more divergent at near than at a distance. This is evidence of:**
    a) Convergence insufficiency
    b) Abnormal retinal correspondence
    c) An intermittent deviation
    d) Amblyopia

19. **Your patient has an esodeviation that is worse at near than at a distance. This is classified as:**
    a) Convergence insufficiency
    b) Convergence excess
    c) Divergence excess
    d) Divergence insufficiency

20. **A and V patterns are types of horizontal deviations that:**
    a) Vary in up and down gaze
    b) Are associated with audio and visual stimuli
    c) Vary in left and right gaze
    d) Cannot be measured accurately

21. **The most common cause of a V pattern is:**
    a) Underactive IO
    b) Overactive SO   •
    c) Overactive IO
    d) Underactive SO

22. **Which pattern is most common?**
    a) V pattern XT
    b) V pattern ET
    c) A pattern XT
    d) A pattern ET

23. **Anisometropia at birth is more likely to result in:**
    a) Esophoria
    b) Esotropia
    c) Exophoria
    d) Exotropia

24. **All of the following are commonly associated with horizontal deviations** *except*:
    a) Adult-onset blindness in one eye
    b) Down's syndrome
    c) Amblyopia
    d) Blow-out fracture of the orbit

25. **Vertical deviations are conventionally described by indicating:**
    a) The higher eye
    b) The lower eye
    c) The preferred eye
    d) The eye with best vision

26. **Decreased elevation of one eye may be due to all of the following *except*:**
    a) Duane's syndrome
    b) Brown's syndrome
    c) Blow-out fracture
    d) Grave's disease

27. **Patients with a new vertical deviation will complain of double vision where the images:**
    a) Are one above or diagonal to the other
    b) Are beside each other
    c) Seem to vibrate
    d) Have a halo around them

28. **In pseudostrabismus:**
    a) The eye turns only if fusion is disrupted
    b) The eyes are straight, but there is amblyopia
    c) The eyes are straight, but the patient has diplopia
    d) The eyes look crossed, but actually are straight

29. **Pseudostrabismus usually is seen in:**
    a) Boys
    b) Girls
    c) Infants
    d) Adults

30. **Pseudoesotropia most often is caused by:**
    a) A flat nasal bridge and epicanthal folds
    b) Hyperthyroidism
    c) A long nose and ptosis
    d) Facial asymmetry

31. **An incomitant deviation, such as occurs in paralytic strabismus:**
    a) Is the same in upgaze as in downgaze
    b) Is the same in right gaze as in left gaze
    c) Is the same in every field of gaze
    d) Varies depending on the field of gaze

32. **The most common patient complaint in a new nerve palsy is:**
    a) Decreased vision
    b) Diplopia
    c) An ache in the affected muscle(s)
    d) An inability to read at near

33. **Nerve palsies cause the affected muscle(s) to become:**
    a) Overactive
    b) Underactive
    c) Spasmodic
    d) Responsive

34. **In order to determine that a new strabismus is paralytic, one should test:**
    a) Vergences
    b) Versions
    c) Ductions
    d) Binocularity

35. **In paralytic strabismus, the measurement taken with the patient fixating with the affected eye is:**
    a) The same as the measurement taken with the patient fixating with the unaffected eye
    b) Greater than the measurement taken with the patient fixating with the unaffected eye
    c) Less than the measurement taken with the patient fixating with the unaffected eye
    d) The only one that is truly accurate

36. **The measurement described in the above question refers to:**
    a) The presence of an A or V pattern
    b) The primary deviation
    c) The secondary deviation
    d) The tertiary deviation

37. **If the deviation described above is measured using the unaffected eye to fixate, the measurement is referred to as:**
    a) An A pattern
    b) The primary deviation
    c) The secondary deviation
    d) A V pattern

38. **The gaze most affected by a palsy of the LR is:**
    a) Abduction
    b) Adduction
    c) Down and in
    d) Up and out

39. **The gaze most affected by a palsy of the SO is:**
    a) Abduction
    b) Adduction
    c) Down and in
    d) Up and out

40. **A common deviation found following head trauma is:**
    a) Bilateral SO palsy
    b) Bilateral LR palsy
    c) Bilateral IO palsy
    d) Bilateral IR palsy

41. **The Bielschowsky 3 step test (B3ST) is used in vertical deviations to:**
    a) Shorten the recovery period
    b) Identify which cyclovertical muscle is at fault
    c) Measure the primary and secondary deviations
    d) Differentiate between an A and V pattern

42. **The B3ST will be accurate in which of the following cases?**
    a) When the patient has had a LR recession
    b) A long-standing muscle palsy
    c) A muscle palsy of recent onset
    d) An orbital floor fracture

43. **Step 1 of the B3ST involves:**
    a) Determining which eye has the best vision
    b) Determining which eye is hypertropic in primary position
    c) Determining which eye is hypotropic in primary position
    d) Determining if the hypertropia is worse in left or right gaze

44. **Step 2 of the B3ST involves:**
    a) Determining which eye is hypertropic in primary position
    b) Determining if the hypertropia is worse in up or down gaze
    c) Determining which eye is hypotropic in primary position
    d) Determining if the hypertropia is worse in left or right gaze

45. **Step 3 of the B3ST involves:**
    a) Determining if the hypertropia is worse in left or right gaze
    b) Determining if the hypertropia is worse in head tilt left or right
    c) Determining if the hypertropia is worse in head turn left or right
    d) Determining if the hypertropia is worse in up or down gaze

46. **Which muscle is weak in the following B3ST example?**
    Step 1: RHT
    Step 2: worse in right gaze
    Step 3: worse in left tilt
    a) RIR
    b) RIO
    c) LSO
    d) LIO

47. **The lay term for amblyopia is:**
    a) Walleyed
    b) Lazy eye
    c) Cross-eyed
    d) Pirate eye

48. **Amblyopia may be manifested as:**
    a) An eye that learns to see with a retinal point other than the fovea
    b) Poor vision in one eye that can be improved with lenses
    c) Poor vision in both eyes that can be improved with lenses
    d) Poor vision in a healthy eye that cannot be improved with lenses

49. **Which of the following is *most* likely to develop amblyopia in the right eye?**
    a) A 3-year-old with a refractive error of -3.00 sphere OD and +0.50 sphere OS
    b) A 3-year-old with a refractive error of +4.00 sphere OD and +1.25 sphere OS
    c) A 12-year-old with convergence insufficiency type exodeviation
    d) A 1-year-old with 1 mm of ptosis on the right

50. **All of the following can cause amblyopia *except*:**
    a) Congenital ptosis that covers the pupil
    b) Alternating strabismus
    c) Congenital cataract
    d) Anisometropia

51. **Clinically, amblyopia is diagnosed when the:**
    a) Best corrected vision of each eye differs by two or more acuity lines
    b) Best corrected vision of each eye differs by four or more acuity lines
    c) Uncorrected vision of each eye differs by four or more acuity lines
    d) Patient cannot appreciate binocular/stereoscopic vision

52. **Which of the following is appropriate when testing a preschooler for amblyopia?**
    a) Single Allen cards
    b) Isolated projected figures
    c) A full line of figures
    d) Single E's

53. **A 3-month-old may be tested for amblyopia by any of the following *except*:**
    a) 25 diopter base in test
    b) Rating central, steady, and maintained
    c) Preferential looking technique (PL)
    d) Visual evoked potential (VEP)

54. **The purpose of covering one eye with an occluder for strabismus testing is to:**
    a) Determine if the patient is suppressing
    b) Perform monocular testing
    c) Disrupt fusion
    d) Determine if the patient is malingering

55. **Cover testing can be performed even on an infant because:**
    a) It is nonthreatening
    b) It is painless
    c) It is objective
    d) It is brief

56. **Cover testing can be useful in all of the following patients *except*:**
    a) Bilateral aphake
    b) Bilateral pseudophake
    c) The patient with suppression
    d) The monocular patient

57. **The cover/uncover test is used to determine the presence of:**
    a) Phoria vs. a tropia
    b) Amblyopia
    c) Suppression
    d) Stereopsis

58. **The cover/uncover test can also reveal the presence of:**
    a) Eso vs. exo
    b) Vergence insufficiency
    c) Depth perception
    d) Visual acuity

59. **You have covered the patient's right eye. When you uncover it, the right eye moves inward. Now you cover the left eye. When you uncover it, the left eye moves inward. You can deduce that the patient has an:**
   a) Exophoria
   b) Exotropia
   c) Exodeviation
   d) Esodeviation

60. **The patient's vision is 20/20 OD and OS. You cover the patient's right eye and note that when you do so, the left eye moves outward. When you uncover the right eye, neither eye moves. When you cover the left eye, the right eye moves outward. When you uncover the left eye, neither eye moves. This indicates:**
   a) Alternating exotropia
   b) Esophoria
   c) Intermittent esotropia
   d) Alternating esotropia

61. **During the cover/uncover test, if a patient has a phoria, the response of the eye that is *not* covered is to:**
   a) Take up fixation
   b) Move in the same direction as the covered eye
   c) Remain straight
   d) Deviate in or out

62. **The alternate (cross) cover test does *not* reveal:**
   a) Exodeviations
   b) Esodeviations
   c) Hyper deviations
   d) A phoria vs. a tropia

63. **When performing the alternate (cross) cover test, it is important to:**
   a) Momentarily remove the cover from one eye before covering the other
   b) Move the cover rapidly from one eye to the other
   c) Allow the patient to look at the target with both eyes before covering again
   d) Move the cover from one eye to the next every half-second

64. **If there is no movement of either eye during any part of the alternate (cross) cover test, one has determined that:**
   a) The patient is amblyopic in one eye
   b) The eyes are orthophoric
   c) The patient has stereo vision
   d) The patient has equal vision in either eye

65. **You have performed the alternate (cross) cover test and notice that each eye moves inward when uncovered. What is your next step?**
   a) Record exodeviation in the chart
   b) Record exotropia in the chart
   c) Record esodeviation in the chart
   d) Perform a cover/uncover test

66. **The alternate (cross) cover test can be used to measure the size of a deviation if:**
   a) The patient can fuse
   b) The corneal reflex can be seen
   c) It is combined with prisms
   d) Polarized glasses are used

67. **All of the following are true regarding the prism and cover test** *except*:
    a) The prism may be split between the two eyes
    b) The prism must be placed in front of the deviated eye
    c) Prisms may be stacked base-to-base and added together
    d) Alternate (cross) covering is used, not cover/uncover

68. **To properly place the prism to measure deviations:**
    a) The prism apex should point in the same direction as the deviation
    b) The prism apex should point in the opposite direction as the deviation
    c) Always split the amount of prism between the two eyes
    d) Always place the prism over the deviating eye

69. **The endpoint of the prism and cover test is reached when:**
    a) The amount of movement is equal in both eyes
    b) No movement is seen on alternate covering
    c) The patient reports that the target is single
    d) The patient reports that the target is double

70. **When measuring a patient with an RHT, the correcting prism could be placed:**
    a) BO, OD
    b) BU, OD
    c) BD, OS
    d) BD, OD

71. **The deviation of a tropic patient is neutralized with a 10 diopter prism, base out, in front of the right eye and a 5 diopter prism, base out, in front of the left eye. This patient has a:**
    a) 5 diopter ET
    b) 5 diopter XT
    c) 15 diopter XT
    d) 15 diopter ET

72. **The deviation of a tropic patient is neutralized with a 15 diopter prism, base up, in front of the right eye and a 5 diopter prism, base up, in front of the left eye. This patient has a:**
    a) 20 diopter RHT
    b) 20 diopter LHT
    c) 10 diopter RHT
    d) 10 diopter LHT

73. **In the Hirschberg and Krimsky tests, a penlight is used to:**
    a) Enable the patient to fixate
    b) Test pupillary reaction
    c) Create a light reflex
    d) Evaluate muscle movements

74. **When performing the Hirschberg test on an orthophoric patient, the light reflexes will usually appear:**
    a) In the middle of the pupil
    b) Slightly nasal to the pupil's center
    c) Slightly temporal to the pupil's center
    d) At the limbus

75. **You are performing a Hirschberg test. What measurement is indicated in the following (Figure 3-2)?**
    a) 30 prism diopters LXT
    b) 90 prism diopters LET
    c) 90 prism diopters LXT
    d) 45 prism diopters LXT

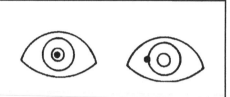

Figure 3-2. Reprinted with permission from Hansen V. *A Systematic Approach to Strabismus*. Thorofare, NJ: SLACK Incorporated; 1998.

76. **You are performing a Hirschberg test. What measurement is indicated in the following (Figure 3-3)?**
    a) 30 prism diopter RET
    b) 60 prism diopter RET
    c) 60 prism diopter RXT
    d) 90 prism diopter RET

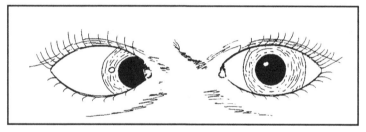

Figure 3-3. Drawing by Holly Hess. From *The Crystal Clear Guide to Sight for Life*. Starburst Publishers. Used by permission.

77. **You are performing a Hirschberg test. What measurement is indicated in the following (Figure 3-4)?**
    a) 30 prism diopter LXT
    b) 30 prism diopter LET
    c) 60 prism diopter LXT
    d) Orthophoria

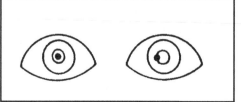

Figure 3-4. Reprinted with permission from Hansen V. *A Systematic Approach to Strabismus*. Thorofare, NJ: SLACK Incorporated; 1998.

78. **The Hirschberg test alone may be appropriate for all of the following situations *except*:**
    a) Bedside examinations
    b) Poorly cooperating infants
    c) Monocular patients
    d) Cooperative binocular patients

79. **The Krimsky measurement combines the Hirschberg method with:**
    a) A prism and cover test
    b) Correcting prisms
    c) A prescription for reading
    d) A Maddox rod

80. **The idea behind the Krimsky measurement is to move the deviated reflex so that:**
    a) There is no movement when you alternate the cover
    b) Both eyes are fixating at the same time
    c) The Hirschberg estimate matches the Krimsky measurement
    d) It falls on the same relative spot as the reflex on the fixating eye

81. **Label the following as: a) Primary, b) Secondary, or c) Tertiary positions of gaze. (Some may be used more than once.)**
    A. Up and right
    B. Straight ahead
    C. Up
    D. Down and left
    E. Up and left
    F. Right
    G. Down and right
    H. Left
    I. Down

82. **Which of the following is *not* considered a cardinal position of gaze?**
    a) Down and left, or up and left
    b) Up and right, or down and right
    c) Straight ahead, or straight up or down
    d) Directly left, or directly right

83. **When testing a patient's versions, it is important to:**
    a) Test in dim lighting
    b) Keep the patient's head still
    c) Use an opaque occluder to break fusion
    d) Keep the patient's eyes in primary position

84. **To test the RIR and the LSO muscles, the patient must look:**
    a) Directly right
    b) Down and to the right
    c) Up and to the right
    d) Down and to the left

85. **Your patient is looking down and to the left. Which muscles are pulling the eyes into this position?**
    a) RIR and LSO
    b) RSO and LIR
    c) RSR and LIO
    d) RIO and LSR

86. **You want to check the action of the RLR. Where do you direct the patient to look?**
    a) To the left
    b) To the right
    c) Down and right
    d) Up and left

87. **You want to check the action of the LIO. Where do you direct the patient to look?**
    a) To the left
    b) Down and right
    c) Up and left
    d) Up and right

88. **The Maddox rod can be used to measure:**
    a) Tropias only
    b) Phorias only
    c) Tropias and phorias
    d) Horizontal deviations only

89. **The Maddox rod test will be accurate in which of the following situations?**
    a) The malingering patient
    b) The patient with suppression
    c) The binocular patient
    d) The monocular patient

90. **The Maddox rod test can be done:**
    a) Only with the eyes in primary gaze
    b) In all fields of gaze
    c) Only at a distance, to avoid accommodation
    d) As an objective measurement

91. **If the Maddox rod is held so that the ridges run up and down, the light coming through it will appear as a:**
    a) Red dot
    b) White dot
    c) Red horizontal line
    d) Red vertical line

92. **You are measuring a patient with a vertical deviation. The Maddox rod should be placed so that the light forms a:**
    a) Horizontal line
    b) Vertical line
    c) Diagonal line
    d) Dot

93. **When measuring a patient with the Maddox rod:**
    a) The correcting prism goes over the Maddox rod
    b) The fixing eye is underneath the Maddox rod
    c) Be sure to use an opaque occluder
    d) Only bar prisms can be used

94. **The endpoint of the Maddox rod test occurs when:**
    a) The red dot is superimposed on the light source
    b) The red line goes through the light
    c) The red line is just above or to the right of the light
    d) The red line disappears

95. **You have placed the Maddox rod before the patient's right eye with the ridges running vertically. Which response would indicate that the patient has a RET?**
    a) The line is to the left of the light
    b) The line is to the right of the light
    c) The line is above the light
    d) None of the above

96. **You have placed the Maddox rod before the patient's left eye with the ridges running horizontally. The patient states that the line is to the right of the light. This indicates:**
    a) LET
    b) LXT
    c) LHT
    d) None of the above

97. **The situation described above is an example of:**
    a) Crossed diplopia
    b) Uncrossed diplopia
    c) A vertical deviation
    d) Suppression

98. **In the situation described above, one would place the prism:**
    a) Base up
    b) Base down
    c) Base out
    d) Base in

99. **The Worth 4 dot (W4D) test is used to determine all of the following *except*:**
    a) Suppression and fusion
    b) Fusional amplitudes
    c) Crossed or uncrossed diplopia
    d) Vertically displaced diplopia

100. **In order for a patient to be able to perform the W4D test, he must:**
    a) Have normal color vision
    b) Be able to interpret his responses
    c) Be able to count objects
    d) Be able to read

101. **The test screen or flashlight used in the W4D test has:**
    a) Four white lights
    b) Two green, one red, and one white light
    c) One green, one red, and two white lights
    d) One green, two red, and one white light

102. **The W4D flashlight should normally be held with:**
    a) The white light on bottom
    b) The red light on bottom
    c) The green light on bottom
    d) A red light to left and right

103. **With the red lens over the right eye, a patient with fusion will report seeing:**
    a) Three lights
    b) Four lights
    c) Five lights
    d) Six lights

104. **A patient with fusion might report all of the following on W4D testing** *except*:
    a) The bottom light switches back and forth from red to green
    b) Only the top light is red, the rest are green
    c) Only the bottom light is red, the rest are green
    d) The top and bottom lights are red, and the left and right lights are green

105. **With the red lens over the right eye during W4D testing, the patient reports seeing only two red lights. This represents:**
    a) Crossed diplopia
    b) Uncrossed diplopia
    c) A vertical deviation
    d) Suppression OS

106. **The patient reports seeing five lights on the W4D test. Your next question should be:**
    a) Do you see all red lights, then all green lights?
    b) Are the red lights on the right side?
    c) Are the red lights on the left side?
    d) Are the red lights above the green lights?

107. **With the red lens over the right eye during W4D testing, the patient reports that there are two red lights to the left of three green lights, indicating:**
    a) Suppression OD
    b) Malingering
    c) Crossed diplopia
    d) No deviation present

108. **In the example above, the deviation present is a(n):**
    a) Esodeviation
    b) Exodeviation
    c) Malingering
    d) Suppression

109. **Stereopsis is recorded in:**
    a) Snellen fractions
    b) Degrees of arc
    c) Seconds of arc
    d) Degrees of field

110. **Bifoveal stereopsis is defined as:**
    a) 20/20
    b) Better than 67 seconds of arc
    c) Better than 45 degrees of arc
    d) Better than 10 degrees of arc

111. **Which of the following indicates the better stereo vision?**
    a) 50 degrees of arc
    b) 25 degrees of arc
    c) 50 seconds of arc
    d) 25 seconds of arc

112. **Stereopsis can be measured in which of the following patients?**
    a) 60 diopter ET
    b) 45 diopter XT
    c) 8 diopter intermittent XT
    d) Monocular

113. **Stereopsis differs from depth perception in that:**
    a) Depth perception is monocular or binocular
    b) Stereo vision involves judging spatial relationships
    c) Depth perception involves seeing in three dimensions
    d) Stereopsis is a learned experience

114. **While it does not give a measurement, a simple stereo test that can be done at bedside is the:**
    a) Hirschberg test
    b) Confrontation stereo test
    c) Pencil point to pencil point test
    d) Amsler grid stereo test

115. **The Titmus test, random dot E, Randot test, and AO distance vectograph slide all utilize:**
    a) Polaroid glasses
    b) Glasses with one red and one green lens
    c) Dissociating prisms
    d) A red filter

116. **You ask a cooperative 3-year-old to touch the wings of the Titmus fly. She recoils and refuses. You can assume that most likely:**
    a) She is tired and cranky
    b) She does not fuse
    c) She does fuse
    d) She has an intermittent deviation

117. **You are testing an intelligent 12-year-old with the Titmus dots, and suspect that he is either a good guesser or a cheater. You should:**
    a) Turn the test 90 degrees
    b) Turn the test 180 degrees
    c) Switch the glasses around
    d) Record the patient's responses regardless

118. **An advantage of the random dot E test over the Titmus test is that the random dot E:**
    a) Does not require special glasses
    b) Offers monocular clues
    c) Does not offer monocular clues
    d) Does not require color vision

119. **The near point of convergence (NPC) is reached when:**
    a) A test object gets so close that one eye deviates inward
    b) A test object gets so close that one eye deviates outward
    c) A test object gets so close that it blurs
    d) A test object is so far away that one eye deviates inward

120. **Judging the NPC by having the patient report diplopia may not always be accurate because the patient might be:**
    a) Amblyopic
    b) Accommodating
    c) Suppressing
    d) Monocular

121. **Which of the following is required in order to perform the NPC test?**
    a) At least 20/40 vision
    b) Depth perception
    c) Normal color vision
    d) Normal fusion

122. **Which of the following regarding NPC is *not* true?**
    a) It tends to become more remote with age
    b) It is more remote with children vs. adults
    c) It is more remote in convergence insufficiency
    d) It can be tested objectively and subjectively

123. **The near point of accommodation (NPA) measures the:**
    a) Amount of bifocal add the patient requires
    b) Distance at which fusion breaks
    c) Distance at which an object doubles
    d) Diopters available for accommodation

124. **To test the NPA:**
    a) Small print is brought closer until it blurs
    b) Small print is brought closer until it doubles
    c) Plus lenses are added until the print clears
    d) A penlight is brought closer until its image blurs

125. **The most accurate way to measure NPA is to:**
    a) Use distant vision correction only in hyperopes
    b) Have the patient wear full distance correction
    c) Have the patient wear full near correction
    d) Correct every patient with a +2.50 lens

126. **NPA should be measured:**
    a) With both eyes together
    b) Separately for each eye
    c) Only if the patient has fusion
    d) Only if the patient has depth perception

127. **Your patient is a fully corrected 30-year-old myope. With glasses on, you measure his NPA, OD, to be 12 cm. This translates to:**
    a) 0.12 diopters
    b) 8.00 diopters
    c) 12.00 diopters
    d) 6.00 diopters

128. **Your patient is a 60-year-old emmetrope with +2.50 reading glasses. You test his NPA, OS, with the readers on, and measure 28.5 cm. What is his available accommodation *without* his readers?**
    a) 1.00 diopters
    b) 2.50 diopters
    c) 3.50 diopters
    d) 6.00 diopters

129. **Ductions refer to:**
    a) Muscles that work against each other during eye movements
    b) Movements of one eye
    c) Movements of both eyes in the same direction
    d) Movements of both eyes in the opposite direction

130. **Testing ductions is useful in differentiating cases of:**
    a) Restrictive strabismus
    b) Accommodative strabismus
    c) Congenital esotropia
    d) Pseudostrabismus

131. **All of the following muscles take part in ductions *except*:**
    a) Agonist
    b) Antagonist
    c) Synergist
    d) Yoke

132. **Versional movements are those which:**
    a) Result in fusion
    b) Move one eye
    c) Move both eyes in the same direction
    d) Move both eyes in a different direction

133. **Version testing evaluates:**
    a) How well a pair of yoke muscles work together
    b) Over and under action of antagonists
    c) How well synergists and agonists work together
    d) Under and over action of an agonist

134. **If the eyes have normal version movements, all of the following will exist *except*:**
    a) Each eye will move with equal speed
    b) Each eye will move smoothly
    c) The eyes will diverge equally
    d) Each eye will be at the same position with respect to the other

135. **Prism and cover testing in a head tilt position is done to evaluate:**
    a) Horizontal deviations
    b) Vertical deviations
    c) Accommodative deviations
    d) A and V patterns

136. **When performing a prism and cover test in a head tilt position, the bottom edge of the prism should:**
    a) Remain parallel to the floor
    b) Be turned perpendicular to the floor
    c) Be turned 90 degrees opposite the head tilt
    d) Remain parallel to the floor of the orbit

137. **The patient tilts her head to the right. The compensatory muscle movements are:**
    a) RIO and RIR extort; LSR and LSO intort
    b) RIO and RIR intort; LSR and LSO extort
    c) RSR and RSO intort; LIO and LIR extort
    d) RSR and RSO extort; LIO and LIR intort

138. **In the Bielschowsky head tilt test:**
    a) A and V patterns are evaluated
    b) Hypertropia with head tilted right, then left, is measured
    c) Hypotropia with head tilted right, then left, is measured
    d) The horizontal deviation with head tilted right, then left, is measured

139. **A compensatory head tilt is most often adopted when the muscle involved is a(n):**
    a) Rectus muscle
    b) Inferior muscle
    c) Superior muscle
    d) Oblique muscle

140. **Your child patient has an abnormal head position. In order to help determine if this is due to strabismus, you should:**
    a) Move the child's head further in that direction, watching for a change in alignment
    b) Move the child's head in the opposite direction, watching for a change in alignment
    c) Move the child's head into primary position and ask if diplopia occurs
    d) Move the child's head into primary position and see how long she maintains it

141. **The compensatory head posture of a patient with a RSO palsy would most likely be:**
    a) Head tilt left and up
    b) Head tilt left and down
    c) Head tilt right and up
    d) Head tilt right and down

142. **Vergence testing examines the ability of the eyes:**
    a) To move in opposite directions in order to maintain stereopsis as an object moves closer or farther away
    b) To move in opposite directions to maintain fixation as an object moves closer or farther away
    c) To move together in the same direction to maintain fixation as an object moves closer or farther away
    d) To judge spatial relationships as an object moves closer or farther away

143. **You are standing at your mailbox waiting for the postman. He drives past you without stopping. As you watch his truck fade in the distance, your eyes are:**
    a) Converging
    b) Diverging
    c) Accommodating
    d) Decompensating

144. **Convergence is linked to:**
   a) Accommodation
   b) Vertical strabismus
   c) Blink rate
   d) Vertical head movements

145. **When vergences are measured, it is important to:**
   a) Measure convergence first, and measure near first
   b) Measure convergence first, and measure distance first
   c) Measure divergence first, and measure near first
   d) Measure divergence first, and measure distance first

146. **To test divergence, the prism is placed:**
   a) Base up
   b) Base down
   c) Base out
   d) Base in

147. **In vergence testing, stronger prism is added until:**
   a) The patient reports the images are superimposed
   b) The patient reports that one image is above the other
   c) The patient reports seeing two images
   d) The patient reports feeling his eyes pull and strain

148. **You are testing divergence and the patient is looking at a 20/40 letter. The patient reports "breaking" at 20 diopters. You should:**
   a) Ask him if he can pull the images together
   b) Record 20 diopters as the breaking point
   c) Show the patient 25 diopters and ask if there are still two images
   d) Tell the patient to close one eye and see if there are still two images

149. **Once the breaking point is found:**
   a) The test is over and the result recorded
   b) Introduce larger prism and ask if the images are still doubled
   c) Introduce smaller prism until the images are fused
   d) Remove the prism and measure the time it takes for the patient to recover

150. **The power of a Risley prism is changed by:**
   a) Moving the prism bar up or down
   b) Putting down one prism and picking up another
   c) Rotating the prism itself
   d) Turning a thumbscrew

151. **An advantage of using the Risley prism is:**
   a) Patients find it more comfortable
   b) It provides a continuous unbroken change in prism power
   c) It increases fusion
   d) It can be used to measure accommodative ability

152. **The red glass test can be used:**
   a) To test cyclodeviations
   b) In the diagnostic positions of gaze
   c) Only in primary position
   d) Only for horizontal deviations

153. **As the patient fixates on a light, the red filter is held in front of one eye. If the patient is fusing, she will see:**
    a) A pink light
    b) A white light
    c) A red light
    d) A red light and a white light

154. **You are holding the red filter in front of the patient's left eye, and she says that she sees only a single white light. This indicates:**
    a) Suppression, OD
    b) Suppression, OS
    c) Crossed diplopia
    d) Uncrossed diplopia

155. **You are holding the red filter in front of the patient's right eye, and he says that he sees a red light to the right of a white light. You will now:**
    a) Record that the patient is malingering
    b) Add base in prism until the images are superimposed
    c) Add base out prism until the images are superimposed
    d) Remove the filter and ask if the patient now sees two white lights

156. **Normal retinal correspondence (NRC) is the situation in which:**
    a) One eye uses the fovea and the other eye does not
    b) One eye suppresses the image
    c) The brain can fuse the images from each fovea
    d) A patient with a deviation uses the fovea of each eye

157. **Abnormal retinal correspondence (ARC) may evolve:**
    a) As an adaptation to strabismus
    b) As an adaptation to presbyopia
    c) As an adaptation to pseudostrabismus
    d) As an adaptation to a phoria

158. **In a patient with ARC:**
    a) Depth perception does not exist
    b) Fine stereo vision exists
    c) Gross fusion may exist
    d) Accommodation is increased

159. **In a patient with ARC, the images:**
    a) Fall on both foveae and are grossly fused
    b) Fall on the fovea of one eye and on a nonfoveal point in the other eye
    c) Fall on nonfoveal points of each eye
    d) Fall on the fovea of one eye and are suppressed by the other eye

160. **An advantage to the Bagolini test is that:**
    a) It requires no special equipment
    b) It is the least dissociating of all the fusion tests
    c) It can differentiate between a phoria and a tropia
    d) It is accurate even in infants

161. **The Bagolini lenses are placed in a trial frame so that:**
    a) One lens is at axis 135 and the other at axis 045
    b) One lens is at axis 090 and the other at axis 045
    c) Both lenses are set at axis 045
    d) Both lenses are set at axis 090

162. **If a patient has difficulty in telling what she sees during the Bagolini test:**
    a) Ask her if the line is on the left or right
    b) Then she probably is color vision deficient and cannot do the test
    c) Have her draw the pattern that she sees
    d) Discontinue the test because this is a positive response

163. **Your patient has tested orthophoric, and reports seeing a cross during the Bagolini test. This means that:**
    a) He is malingering
    b) He has ARC
    c) He has NRC
    d) He has a phoria

164. **Your patient has tested esotropic, and reports seeing a cross during the Bagolini test. This indicates that:**
    a) She is malingering
    b) She has NRC
    c) She is fusing
    d) She is not fusing

165. **If your patient has ARC and suppression, the Bagolini targets will appear as:**
    a) A single line
    b) A cross
    c) Two parallel streaks
    d) Two streaks, one with a gap

166. **If your patient has suppression and no binocular vision, he will see:**
    a) A single line
    b) A cross
    c) Two parallel streaks
    d) A line with a gap

Chapter 4

Visual Fields

1. **Each mm on the retina is equal to how many degrees on the visual field?**
   a) 2 degrees
   b) 3 degrees
   c) 4 degrees
   d) 5 degrees

2. **The light receptor cells of the retina are the:**
   a) Retinal pigment epithelium
   b) Rods and cones
   c) Bipolar cells
   d) Ganglion cells

3. **An object on the patient's right will be perceived by the patient's:**
   a) Temporal retina OU
   b) Nasal retina OU
   c) Temporal retina OS and nasal retina OD
   d) Foveae OU

4. **The nerve fibers are axon extensions of the:**
   a) Rods and cones
   b) Ganglion cells
   c) Bipolar layer
   d) Mueller cells

5. **Label the following drawing (Figure 4-1):**
Horizontal raphe	Optic disc
Temporal fibers	Radiating nasal fibers

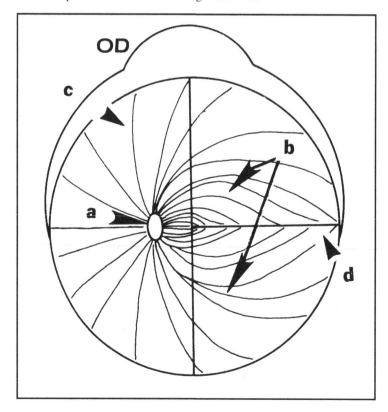

Figure 4-1. Reprinted with permission from Garber N. *Visual Field Examination*. Thorofare, NJ: SLACK Incorporated; 1998.

6. **Label the following illustration (Figure 4-2), which shows the visual field of the right eye and the corresponding retinal nerve fiber distribution.**
   Superior retinal nerve fibers
   Optic disc
   Temporal retinal nerve fibers
   Macula
   Nasal retinal nerve fibers
   Horizontal raphe
   Inferior retinal nerve fibers

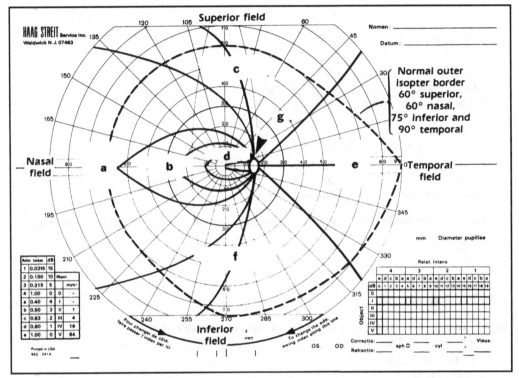

Figure 4-2. Reprinted with permission from Garber N. *Visual Field Examination*. Thorofare, NJ: SLACK Incorporated; 1998.

7. **The anatomic pattern of the nerve fibers produces visual field defects:**
   a) That are total blind spots
   b) That correspond to the location of the rods and cones
   c) That correspond to the location of the nerve fibers
   d) That respond well to treatment

8. **The "blind spot" as plotted on a visual field test corresponds to:**
   a) The macula
   b) The fovea
   c) The optic disk
   d) The lamina cribrosa

9. **The size of the average blind spot is:**
   a) 5.5 degrees wide and 7.5 degrees high
   b) 7.5 degrees wide and 5.5 degrees high
   c) 3.5 degrees wide and 5.5 degrees high
   d) 7.5 degrees wide and 10.5 degrees high

10. **On the visual field, the average blind spot is located:**
    a) 25 degrees temporal to fixation
    b) 5 degrees nasal to fixation
    c) 15 degrees nasal to fixation
    d) 15 degrees temporal to fixation

11. **If you increase the visual field testing distance, the blind spot will:**
    a) Stay the same in both cm and degrees
    b) Get larger in both cm and degrees
    c) Get larger in cm but remain the same in degrees
    d) Stay the same in cm but get larger in degrees

12. **At the chiasm:**
    a) Nerve impulses are magnified before traveling on to the brain
    b) Nerve impulses are sorted before traveling on to the brain
    c) Nasal nerve fibers from each eye cross over to the opposite side
    d) Temporal nerve fibers from each eye cross over to the opposite side

13. **The gland that lies in the chiasmal region and can have a direct impact on the visual field is the:**
    a) Thyroid
    b) Pituitary
    c) Adrenal cortex
    d) Hypothalamus

14. **The characteristic visual field defect due to a lesion at the chiasm is:**
    a) Bitemporal hemianopsia
    b) Binasal hemianopsia
    c) Left hemianopsia
    d) Right hemianopsia

15. **After nerve fibers cross at the chiasm, they pass next through the:**
    a) Lamina cribrosa
    b) Optic tract
    c) Optic radiations
    d) Optic nerve

16. **As the nerve fibers pass through the optic tract, they:**
    a) Intensify the light impulses
    b) Rotate, thus changing position
    c) Cross over to the other side of the brain
    d) Pass under the pituitary gland

17. **After leaving the optic tract, the nerve fibers bundle together at a "relay station" known as the:**
    a) Optic radiations
    b) Optic disk
    c) Visual cortex
    d) Lateral geniculate body

18. **The layers of the lateral geniculate body nucleus are divided so that half of the layers are made up of crossed fibers, and half are made up of uncrossed fibers. How many layers are there?**
    a) Four
    b) Six
    c) Eight
    d) Ten

19. **Which of the following is *not* true regarding the nerve fibers once they exit the lateral geniculate body?**
    a) The tract continues to rotate
    b) They fan out forming the optic radiations
    c) The temporal lobe fibers form Meyer's loop
    d) They enter the brain tissue

20. **Visual nerve fibers terminate at the:**
    a) Brainstem
    b) Occipital cortex
    c) Thalamus
    d) Meyer's loop

21. **Visual field defects become more congruous:**
    a) If both optic nerves are affected
    b) If the intraocular pressure (IOP) in both eyes is elevated
    c) If the lesion is in one eye only
    d) The closer the lesion is to the occipital cortex

22. **Sensory input (light impulses) on the patient's left is transmitted to the:**
    a) Temporal retina OS and nasal retina OD
    b) Left side of each retina
    c) Left optic tract
    d) Right side of the brain

23. **The boundary of an area that responds to the same stimulus intensity is called a(n):**
    a) Isopter
    b) Scotoma
    c) Decibel
    d) Homonymous

24. **An area inside a visual field isopter that does not respond to any of the targets available on that particular machine is termed a:**
    a) Contortion
    b) Constriction
    c) Bjerrum's
    d) Scotoma

25. "At threshold" means that the patient responds to a given stimulus in the same area:
a) 25% of the time
b) 50% of the time
c) 75% of the time
d) 100% of the time

26. An apostilb is a measurement of:
a) Target size
b) Target value
c) Light intensity
d) Target color wavelength

27. The arbitrary decibel unit is used to denote stimulus intensity in:
a) Automated perimetry
b) Goldmann perimetry
c) Tangent screen testing
d) Confrontation visual fields

28. The decibel unit is considered arbitrary because:
a) It may differ from one machine to another
b) It cannot be controlled
c) It depends on the cleanliness of the targets
d) It depends on the minimum available stimulus intensity

29. The decibel scale is dependent on:
a) The maximum intensity of that machine's stimulus
b) Room lighting during visual fields testing
c) The patient's contrast sensitivity
d) The stimulus color

30. The higher the decibel rating:
a) The smaller the target
b) The brighter the light intensity
c) The dimmer the light intensity
d) The higher the threshold

31. Regarding visual field testing, the term *calibration* refers to:
a) Proper selection of the target size
b) Checking the light intensity and adjusting if needed
c) Checking and installing the recording paper
d) Installing the proper bulbs prior to use

32. Matching. Match the term to the correct definition.

Terms:	Definitions:
A. Absolute	a) The central dot on the visual field chart
B. Altitudinal	b) Rings around the center point designated in degrees
C. Bjerrum area	c) Diameter lines designated in degrees
D. Congruous	d) Point where a stimulus is seen 50% of the time
E. Constricted	e) A stimulus that is too small or too dim to be seen
F. Depression	f) A stimulus that exceeds threshold and is seen over 50% of the time
G. Eccentricities	g) Boundary of points with the same sensitivity
H. Fixation	h) Area within an isopter where threshold is not seen

I.	Hemianopsia	i)	Scotoma that is blind to every stimulus
J.	Heteronymous	j)	Scotoma that is sensitive to suprathreshold stimuli
K.	Homonymous	k)	An entire isopter that is moved inward from expected normal
L.	Incongruous	l)	A portion of an isopter that is moved inward from expected normal
M.	Infrathreshold	m)	Constriction of the isopter along the 180 degree meridian
N.	Isopter	n)	Area between the 10 degree and 18 degree eccentricities
O.	Meridians	o)	Defect involving the superior or inferior field
P.	Quadrantanopsia	p)	Defect involving the left or right field
Q.	Relative	q)	Defect involving one fourth of the field of each eye
R.	Scotoma	r)	Defect involving opposite sides of each eye
S.	Step	s)	Defect involving the same side of each eye
T.	Suprathreshold	t)	Defect that looks the same in both eyes
U.	Threshold	u)	Defect that looks different in either eye

33. The extent of vision beyond the fixation point is known as the:

a) Binocular field

b) Visual field

c) Neurological field

d) Visual pathway

34. The peripheral vision of a normal person is:

a) 60 degrees temporal, 60 degrees inferior, 75 degrees nasal, and 95 degrees superior

b) 75 degrees temporal, 60 degrees inferior, 95 degrees nasal, and 60 degrees superior

c) 95 degrees temporal, 60 degrees inferior, 75 degrees nasal, and 60 degrees superior

d) 95 degrees temporal, 75 degrees inferior, 60 degrees nasal, and 60 degrees superior

35. The configuration of the normal visual field is delimited by:

a) The ear and nasal bridge

b) The brow and nose

c) The location of the fovea

d) The size of the optic nerve

36. Conversion of the visual field map into a three-dimensional representation results in:

a) Isopters

b) The island of vision profile

c) A comparative analysis

d) Threshold graytone analysis

37. The peak of the island of vision profile corresponds to the:

a) Optic nerve

b) Center of the crystalline lens

c) Nerve fiber layer

d) Fovea

38. The blind spot would be represented on the island of vision profile as:

a) A bottomless hole

b) A peak

c) A shallow dip

d) A deep pit

39. In the island of vision analogy, vision exists in:
a) A sea of blindness
b) A sea of vision
c) An expanse of vision
d) A time-space continuum

40. In the island of vision analogy, peripheral vision that gradually decreases as it extends outward would be represented by a:
a) Bottomless hole
b) Gentle slope
c) Sharp drop-off
d) Flat area

41. Which of the following is *true* regarding visual field screening techniques?
a) They are difficult for patients because of the time required
b) They are not practical for evaluating large groups
c) Their main purpose is to rule out pathology
d) They cannot be used to confirm changes in prior fields

42. Which of the following is *not* true regarding visual field screening techniques?
a) Always plot the blind spot if the chosen technique permits
b) A defect should be verified by more in-depth testing
c) Limited information is generated
d) The same screening protocol is used for every patient

43. The Harrington-Flocks screener utilizes:
a) A series of test pattern cards and ultraviolet light
b) A black screen and hand held targets
c) A black screen and the examiner's fingers
d) An automated perimeter

44. An automated single intensity screening program determines a few threshold values, extrapolates the individual's island of vision, then:
a) Tests points with a supposed suprathreshold stimulus
b) Runs the test using standardized stimuli for abnormal fields
c) Tests points using a supposed infrathreshold stimulus
d) Plots isopters, gives numerical data, and estimates fluctuation

45. Automated threshold testing:
a) Basically gives a yes/no response
b) Measures sensitivity at each tested point
c) Tests each point with a suprathreshold stimulus
d) Tests each point with a standardized stimulus

46. Accurately determining threshold requires:
a) Using a "normal" threshold as a starting point
b) Moving from seeing to nonseeing
c) A single testing of a point
d) Multiple testing of the same point

47. **A patient might not respond to a suprathreshold stimuli:**
    a) By chance
    b) Because it is too dim
    c) Because it is too small
    d) Because it is too large

48. **The threshold level in kinetic perimetry is affected by:**
    a) The fact that a larger target is necessary
    b) The fact that the target is moving
    c) The fact that the target is stationary
    d) Computer or operator error

49. **Automated threshold tests generally start with a suprathreshold stimulus, then:**
    a) Test all points at that illumination
    b) Increase illumination until the stimulus is not seen, then gradually decrease illumination until the stimulus is seen again
    c) Decrease illumination until the stimulus is not seen and record this as threshold
    d) Decrease illumination until the stimulus is not seen, then gradually increase illumination until the stimulus is seen again

50. **The starting point to determine threshold in an automated perimeter program might come from all of the following *except*:**
    a) Information from the patient's last test
    b) The patient's threshold at several predetermined points
    c) The threshold at the patient's optic nerve
    d) Using age-related normal values

51. **The validity of all visual field testing depends on:**
    a) The technical skill of the operator
    b) The patient's ability to maintain fixation
    c) The complexity of the screening program
    d) The illumination capabilities of the instrument used

52. **The blind spot *cannot* be plotted by which of the following methods?**
    a) Bowl perimeter
    b) Arc perimeter
    c) Amsler grid
    d) Tangent screen

53. **The main challenge in testing the visual fields of low vision patients is:**
    a) Their inability to understand the test
    b) Their inability to see the fixation area
    c) Finding the appropriate threshold
    d) Finding the appropriate correcting lens

54. **Manual perimetry involves testing the visual field:**
    a) At preset points
    b) Using stationary stimuli
    c) Using moving stimuli
    d) Using both stationary and moving stimuli

55. **An advantage to manual perimetry over automated is that manual perimetry:**
    a) Permits testing of preselected points
    b) Permits testing of the entire visual field
    c) Is more accurate with static threshold testing
    d) Is more reproducible

56. **The main disadvantage of manual perimetry is that:**
    a) The entire visual field cannot be tested
    b) It is difficult to locate scotomata
    c) It requires a higher degree of technical skill
    d) Isopters cannot be accurately plotted

57. **What is the given assumption in confrontation field testing?**
    a) The patient has 20/20 vision
    b) The fields are tested in the central area
    c) The examiner's field is normal
    d) The procedure is fully qualitative

58. **The confrontation field:**
    a) Requires the use of elaborate equipment
    b) Will not pick up gross visual field defects
    c) Can be performed on a patient in any position
    d) Cannot be performed on children

59. **Which of the following is *not* true regarding the confrontation visual field test?**
    a) The examiner's back should be toward a blank wall
    b) Only the examiner's fingers should be used as a target
    c) The eye not being tested is occluded
    d) A defect can be either described in words or drawn out in the chart

60. **The tangent screen and Autoplot® are used to map:**
    a) The central 20 degrees
    b) The central 30 degrees
    c) The central 40 degrees
    d) The peripheral field outside 20 degrees

61. **Advantages of the Autoplot® include all of the following *except*:**
    a) Fixation is assisted by use of a chin rest
    b) It is portable
    c) Size and intensity of the test object are easily changed
    d) Testing distance can be varied

62. **If you are using a felt-type tangent screen, patient responses should be marked using:**
    a) A chalk marker
    b) Standard sewing pins
    c) Black-head pins
    d) A pencil

63. **During a tangent screen test the patient should:**
    a) Wear his distant correction
    b) Wear his near correction
    c) Remove all correction
    d) Wear a contact lens if the refractive error is over 3.00 diopters

64. **If you are performing a tangent screen and the patient wears bifocal lenses, the patient should:**
    a) Remove the glasses when you test the inferior field
    b) Tuck her chin so the inferior field is viewed with the distance portion of the lens
    c) Look through the bifocal when you test the inferior field
    d) Remove the glasses for the entire test

65. **When plotting the patient's left field using a tangent screen, the examiner should stand:**
    a) On the patient's left, facing the patient
    b) On the patient's right, facing the patient
    c) On the patient's left, facing the screen
    d) In the center

66. **The correct speed for moving a tangent screen target is approximately:**
    a) 1 degree per second
    b) 5 degrees per second
    c) 10 degrees per second
    d) It doesn't matter as long as the motion is smooth

67. **You look at a patient's previous tangent screen test and see the notation "2/1000 green." This means that:**
    a) A 2 mm green target was used at 1 m
    b) The patient's vision is 2/1000 and his eyes are green
    c) A 2 mm target was used at 1 m and the patient's eyes are green
    d) A 2 mm green target was used at 1000 cm

68. **For a tangent screen test on a 2 x 2 m screen, the patient is usually seated:**
    a) 1000 cm from the screen
    b) 1 m from the screen
    c) 2 m from the screen
    d) 4 m from the screen

69. **Using the tangent screen to confirm a severely contracted field of 5 degrees in a patient suspected of malingering, the patient first is tested with a 3 mm target at 1 m. Then the test is repeated at 2 m using a:**
    a) 1 mm target
    b) 2 mm target
    c) 3 mm target
    d) 6 mm target

70. **An arc perimeter consists of:**
    a) A flat screen and arc-shaped targets
    b) A bowl screen that is rotated in an arc with projected targets
    c) An arc that is rotated, with a target that is moved by hand or mechanically
    d) An arc-shaped screen, and electrodes that are attached to the patient's temples

71. **Arc perimetry is most useful for:**
    a) Plotting outer isopters
    b) Plotting the central 30 degrees
    c) Static perimetry
    d) Static threshold measurements

72. **When testing the patient's right eye on an arc perimeter, the patient's chin should be:**
   a) In the right chin rest
   b) In the left chin rest
   c) In the central chin rest
   d) This instrument has no chin rest

73. **For arc perimetry, the untested eye is patched and the tested eye:**
   a) Wears no correction
   b) Wears habitual near correction
   c) Wears habitual distance correction
   d) Is corrected with a +2.50 sphere

Note: Questions 74-89 refer to Goldmann perimetry.

74. **Advantages of the Goldmann perimeter include all of the following *except*:**
   a) Fixation can be monitored easily
   b) Its portability
   c) Its versatility in kinetic testing
   d) The target can be projected and the chart marked simultaneously

75. **Once the Goldmann perimeter is calibrated, and the patient is educated and positioned, one should:**
   a) Plot the blind spot
   b) Plot the outer isopter with the I4e
   c) Find a threshold starting point
   d) Statically spot-check several points outside the central 30 degrees

76. **Which of the following is correct progression when determining a threshold stimulus to use as a starting point for mapping the outer periphery?**
   a) I2e, I3e, I4e, II4e, II4e, III4e, IV4e, V4e
   b) V4e, IV4e, III4e, II4e, II4e, I4e, I3e, I2e
   c) I2e, II2e, III2e, IV2e, V2e, I3e, II3e, III3e, etc.
   d) I2a, I2b, I2c, I2d, I2e, II2a, II2b, II2c, etc.

77. **Maximum illumination is achieved at the I4e setting. If the patient does *not* respond to this stimulus:**
   a) One cannot perform a Goldmann on this patient
   b) Use a +3.00 add for the entire test
   c) Have the patient sit 1 m back from the bowl and try again
   d) Increase the target size

78. **The outer isopter should be mapped with the threshold stimulus found:**
   a) At central fixation
   b) Within the central 30 degrees
   c) 15 degrees temporal to fixation
   d) 50 degrees temporal to fixation

79. **If the patient is having a follow-up visual field:**
   a) Use threshold stimuli as determined on this date
   b) Use the same stimuli as the last test
   c) Use a stimulus 1 degree brighter or larger than the last test
   d) Use a stimulus 1 degree dimmer or smaller than the last test

80. **If the patient has poor vision and is having trouble seeing the fixation area in the Goldmann bowl:**
    a) The mirror inside the viewing port should be put in place
    b) Use a +3.00 add for the entire test
    c) Have the patient wear her glasses
    d) Put a cross of black tape over the fixation area to enlarge it

81. **The central field is tested and mapped inside which eccentricity?**
    a) 5 degrees
    b) 15 degrees
    c) 30 degrees
    d) 90 degrees

82. **To find a suitable stimulus for mapping the central field, determine the threshold:**
    a) Of central fixation
    b) 15 degrees temporal to fixation
    c) 25 degrees temporal to fixation
    d) Two "notches" dimmer than that used for the outermost isopter

83. **For kinetic perimetry, the Goldmann stimulus should be moved:**
    a) Smoothly at 5 degrees per second
    b) In an oscillatory motion at 5 degrees per second
    c) In a straight line at 1 degree per second
    d) Around the eccentricities at 10 degrees per second

84. **In general, mapping out isopters and scotomas is accomplished by:**
    a) Moving the stimulus from seeing to nonseeing
    b) Moving the stimulus from nonseeing to seeing
    c) Presenting a stationary stimulus for a yes/no response
    d) Moving the stimulus from left to right

85. **Difficulty in finding the blind spot may be due to all of the following *except*:**
    a) Failure to patch the opposite eye
    b) Enlarged blind spot due to glaucoma
    c) A stimulus that is too large or moved too fast
    d) Fixation loss

86. **When plotting the isopter at 90 degrees, 0 degrees, and 180 degrees:**
    a) Plot the isopter at 30 degree intervals
    b) Plot the isopter directly at 90, 0, and 180, plus 15 degrees on either side
    c) Plot the isopter at 5 and 15 degrees to either side
    d) Plot the isopter every 5 degrees for 30 degrees on either side

87. **If a constriction or scotoma is detected:**
    a) Continue using only standard examination technique
    b) Map the defect with at least two different targets
    c) Map the defect only with the stimulus with which it was detected
    d) Introduce a +3.00 add and see how the defect size changes

88. **You are mapping the nasal field, OD, with a I4e target. On the 175 degree meridian, the target appears at the 60 degree eccentricity. On the 150 degree meridian, the target appears at the 30 degree eccentricity. You should:**
    a) Connect the points with a line
    b) Check the 195 degree meridian
    c) Bring the stimulus perpendicularly between the two points
    d) Use a brighter or larger target that will extend the isopter

89. **Fixation monitoring on the Goldmann perimeter:**
    a) Can be done continuously through the viewer port
    b) Can be done even with the fixation mirror in place
    c) Is done only when testing the blind spot
    d) Is adequate if checked once every 5 minutes

    Note: Questions 90-101 are all concerning automated perimetry.

90. **In automated perimetry, stimuli are presented at specific locations. Which of the following is *not* true?**
    a) Test accuracy depends on the density of the test points and the retina's sensitivity at those points
    b) If tested points are spaced 6 degrees apart, a scotoma the size of the blind spot could be missed
    c) All tests are based on a 120 point system
    d) Tested locations are usually placed on meridians and eccentricities

91. **The smallest size pupil diameter allowable for adequate mapping of the periphery is:**
    a) 1 mm
    b) 3 mm
    c) 5 mm
    d) 7 mm

92. **Matching. Match the computer related terms to their definitions.**

Terms:	Definitions:
A. Back up	a) Computer viewing screen
B. Default	b) Used to enter data into the computer
C. Field	c) Spaces where specific information is to be entered
D. Formatting	d) A list of options
E. Keyboard	e) The switch that tells the computer to enter data
F. Menu	f) Preparing a computer disk to receive information
G. Monitor	g) A duplicate disk copy
H. Parameters	h) A setting that is programmed to be used automatically unless specifically changed
I. Point array	i) The selection of points that are tested
J. Return or enter key	j) The variables that can be introduced into the test

93. **Maintenance measures for automated perimeters include all of the following *except*:**
    a) A surge protector for the electrical outlet
    b) Initializing (formatting) the hard drive once a week
    c) Using anti-static spray on carpeted surfaces around the instrument
    d) Covering the instrument when not in use

94. **Target exposure time on an automated perimeter is usually:**
    a) 0.1 to 0.4 seconds
    b) 0.5 to 0.7 seconds
    c) 0.9 to 1.0 seconds
    d) 1.0 to 1.5 seconds

95. **Threshold is dependent on all of the following *except*:**
    a) Background and stimulus intensity
    b) The patient's age
    c) The patient's level of stereopsis
    d) Distance of stimulus from the fovea

96. **Decreasing the illumination of the background:**
    a) Increases the visibility of the target
    b) Decreases the visibility of the target
    c) Means that a smaller target can be used
    d) Decreases contrast

97. **If the patient has poor vision and cannot see the fixation target in the center of the automated perimeter:**
    a) Activate an eccentric fixation pattern
    b) Turn off the fixation monitoring option
    c) Increase the size of the stimulus
    d) Use a +3.00 correcting lens to provide magnification

98. **In order for a threshold point to be considered abnormal:**
    a) It must fall outside the 95th percentile for normal patients
    b) It must be consistently measured as >50 dB
    c) It must be consistently measured as <10 dB
    d) It must be seen 50% of the time

99. **A "normal" screening test means that:**
    a) The patient has no visual field defect
    b) The patient has no field defect detectable by this test
    c) Confrontation visual fields are adequate for future testing
    d) The patient does not have glaucoma

100. **Which of the following is *not* true regarding test results found with an automated perimeter?**
    a) The data can be rearranged into a variety of printouts
    b) It is valid only if the same person performs the test each time
    c) The data can be compared with the patient's previous test(s)
    d) The data can be compared to normal age-related values

101. **When comparing automated fields from one instrument to that of another, it is important to remember that:**
    a) Some automated instruments use projected stimuli while others use light-emitting diodes (LEDs)
    b) Automated instruments vary in their stimulus and background intensity
    c) The correcting lens used should be the same in order to make a fair comparison
    d) Some instruments do not require a lens to correct for near

102. **Moving a target across a screen or other surface from a point where it is not seen to a point where the patient responds is known as:**
    a) Static perimetry
    b) Kinetic perimetry
    c) Threshold perimetry
    d) Formal perimetry

103. **Using stationary targets to measure a retinal receptor's ability to detect the stimulus is known as:**
    a) Static perimetry
    b) Kinetic perimetry
    c) Automated perimetry
    d) Threshold perimetry

104. **For the most part, the technique used by automated perimeters is:**
    a) Static perimetry
    b) Kinetic perimetry
    c) Confrontation perimetry
    d) Decibel designations

105. **Kinetic perimetry can be employed in all of the following techniques *except*:**
    a) Tangent screen
    b) Harrington-Flocks
    c) Arc perimeter
    d) Confrontation fields

106. **Using static perimetry to measure a retinal receptor's threshold is actually a function of the receptor's:**
    a) Color vision
    b) Cone cell concentration
    c) Rod cell concentration
    d) Contrast sensitivity

107. **If you desire to generate a map of the island of vision from the top-down, as if you are hovering over it, the test modality you should choose is:**
    a) Kinetic perimetry
    b) Static perimetry
    c) Threshold perimetry
    d) Automated perimetry

108. **Static perimetry is analogous to:**
    a) Viewing the island of vision from above
    b) Shooting harpoons into the island from the same height all the way around the island
    c) Cutting a horizontal slice through the island of vision
    d) Dropping a paratrooper onto one spot on the island of vision

109. **Which of the following is the more sensitive test?**
    a) Kinetic perimetry
    b) Threshold static perimetry
    c) Suprathreshold static perimetry
    d) Kinetic perimetry with a red target

110. **Regarding calibration of the Goldmann perimeter:**
    a) The bulb and background reflectance should be calibrated daily prior to use
    b) The bulb and background reflectance should be calibrated and adjusted for each patient
    c) The bulb should be calibrated daily and the background reflectance adjusted for each patient
    d) The bulb should be calibrated weekly and the background reflectance should be adjusted daily

111. **Calibration is required to make sure that the Goldmann perimeter's maximum projected light is:**
    a) 100 asbs
    b) 500 asbs
    c) 1000 asbs
    d) 5000 asbs

112. **The background illumination of the Goldmann perimeter should be set to:**
    a) 31.5 asbs
    b) 35.1 asbs
    c) 45.5 asbs
    d) 50.1 asbs

113. **During stimulus calibration of the Goldmann perimeter, the filter levers are set at:**
    a) I4e
    b) II2b
    c) I1a
    d) V4e

114. **If the Goldmann stimulus does not register at 1000 asbs, you either need to replace the bulb or:**
    a) Replace the fuse and remeasure
    b) Lower the background light to compensate
    c) Increase the background light to compensate
    d) Rotate the bulb 180 degrees and remeasure

115. **When setting the background illumination of the Goldmann perimeter, the filter levers should be set at:**
    a) I4e
    b) V4e
    c) V1e
    d) II2b

116. **In order to adjust the background illumination of the Goldmann perimeter to the proper level:**
    a) Slide the shield until the luminescence of bowl and target are equal
    b) Rotate the housing screw until the bowl luminescence is just above that of the target
    c) Slide the shield until the scale reads 35.1
    d) Slide the shield until the scale reads 31.5

117. **At the beginning of each day before using an automated perimeter:**
    a) The background reflectance must be calibrated
    b) The stimulus illumination must be calibrated
    c) The technician should run a diagnostic test
    d) Check the amount of printer paper in the machine

118. **Decreased bulb brightness in an automated visual field machine may be indicated by:**
    a) The instrument's failure to power up
    b) Threshold values other than <0
    c) Failure to find the blind spot
    d) Unexplained field contraction

119. **The visual field chart should include all of the following** *except*:
    a) Patient name, diagnosis, vision, and date
    b) Pupil size, refraction, and near add used for central 30 degrees
    c) Patient's fixation, cooperation, and validity
    d) Objective responses of the patient

120. **The Goldmann visual field chart is traditionally:**
    a) Marked with checks and x's in lead pencil
    b) Color coded to indicate the size and intensity of the stimulus
    c) Grayscale coded to indicate the size and intensity of the stimulus
    d) Automatically created by the pantograph

121. **If the patient's responses are inconsistent in a certain area, this can be indicated on the Goldmann perimeter chart by:**
    a) Plotting as a definite isopter or border using your best judgment
    b) Moving the target faster and plotting as a definite isopter labeled "faster"
    c) Drawing a crosshatch in that area and labeling it as "in and out"
    d) Such an area should not be plotted or reported

122. **Points that are statically spot-checked for scotomas on the Goldmann perimeter:**
    a) May be indicated by coding that isopter with a color indicating stimulus size and intensity
    b) Need not be marked on the chart as long as you do the test the same way every time
    c) May be indicated by filling in that section on the grid, color coded to the stimulus size and intensity
    d) May be indicated by a small mark, color coded to the stimulus size and intensity

123. **Regarding data entry on an automated perimeter:**
    a) One may use all the data from a previous test
    b) The computer automatically makes changes from one test to another
    c) The computer automatically saves displayed data, even if the machine is shut off
    d) It must be entered in the prescribed manner or the computer will not find it later

124. **All of the following are true regarding computer data disks** *except*:
    a) They are sensitive to magnetic fields
    b) They should be left in the computer at all times
    c) An extra copy should be stored apart from the testing site
    d) A log book should be kept to cross-reference files

125. **The numeric pattern (value table) printout for an automated field:**
    a) Displays a threshold using symbols on a grid that corresponds to the test points
    b) Displays probability on a grid that corresponds to the test points
    c) Displays the decibel threshold on a grid that corresponds to the test points
    d) Displays the apostilb threshold on a grid that corresponds to the test points

126. **On the numeric printout of an automated field, the number zero indicates that:**
    a) The stimulus was seen 100% of the time
    b) The stimulus was infrathreshold
    c) The dimmest stimulus was used
    d) The brightest stimulus was not seen

127. **A gray scale printout for automated fields:**
   a) Displays the threshold decibel measurements as a graphic display of varying shades
   b) Displays an "x" if the target was seen and an "o" if the target was not seen
   c) Displays the probability of a normal person seeing that point as a graphic display of varying shades
   d) Displays the differences of the patient's current test to a previous test using a graphic display of varying shades

128. **A point that is not seen is represented on a grayscale printout by:**
   a) A white area
   b) A dot
   c) A black area
   d) An x

129. **To get the best grayscale printout on a computerized field, the technician must test in which modality?**
   a) Suprathreshold single stimulus
   b) Three-zone test
   c) Comprehensive threshold
   d) Hill of vision profile

130. **The depth of defect automated printout:**
   a) Compares the patient's results to expected results
   b) Gives the threshold values of defects in dB
   c) Gives the threshold values of defects in apostilbs
   d) Shows the isopters' defects

131. **The comparison printout on an automated perimeter is designed to:**
   a) Compare the patient's results to normal
   b) Compare the patient's test with and without a correcting lens
   c) Compare the patient's current results to a previous test
   d) Compare the patient's responses to one stimulus with another

132. **A notation of -2 on a point from a comparison printout means:**
   a) The previous test was 2 dB lower than the present test
   b) A loss of 2 dB from the previous test to the present
   c) That particular point has a threshold less than 2 dB
   d) The patient had two varying responses for that point

133. **A correcting lens is required to test:**
   a) Presbyopic patients
   b) Every patient
   c) Hyperopic patients only
   d) On a patient-by-patient basis

134. **The area of the field that is tested by using a near add is:**
   a) The central 20 degrees
   b) The central 30 degrees
   c) The foveal area
   d) The blind spot

135. The best type of lens to use for the near add is:
   a) The patient's own glasses
   b) A lens from any trial lens set
   c) Spheres only
   d) A lens with a thin rim

136. If the patient's distance correction is over + 10.00 D:
   a) A contact lens is required to do the test
   b) Field landmarks will be displaced
   c) A trial lens is required for the entire test
   d) There is no difference from any other field test

137. The visual field in a high hyperope will be:
   a) Compressed, with a blind spot closer to fixation than normal
   b) Expanded, with a blind spot farther from fixation than normal
   c) Compressed, with a smaller blind spot than normal
   d) Expanded, with a larger blind spot than usual

138. A high myope will have a field that is:
   a) Compressed, with a blind spot closer to fixation than normal
   b) Expanded, with a blind spot farther from fixation than normal
   c) Compressed, with a smaller blind spot than normal
   d) Expanded, with a larger blind spot than usual

139. When calculating the near add for visual field testing:
   a) Cylinder amounts under 1.00 D can be ignored
   b) Cylinder amounts over 1.00 D are incorporated as a spherical equivalent
   c) Cylinder amounts are incorporated as a spherical equivalent regardless of amount
   d) Cylinder amounts under 1.00 D are incorporated as a spherical equivalent

140. An emmetropic patient who is 35 years old:
   a) Requires no near add for central fields
   b) Requires a -0.50 D add for central fields
   c) Requires a +1.00 add for central fields
   d) Requires an add only if dilated

141. Calculation of the correcting lens for visual fields (300 mm test distance) in an ametropic patient:
   a) Uses the distance prescription plus the power of the patient's habitual add
   b) Uses the distance prescription without any add
   c) Starts with the distance prescription, then uses an add related to the patient's age
   d) Uses the power of the patient's add without regard to any distance correction

142. In a fully dilated emmetropic patient, which near add correction is required to test the central field?
   a) None
   b) +1.25 D
   c) +2.00 D
   d) +3.25 D

143. **Calculation of the add for automated perimetry includes the factors of:**
   a) Full distance correction and age-related add
   b) Full distance correction and habitual add
   c) Full distance correction, age-related add, and bowl depth
   d) Full distance correction and a 30 cm bowl depth

144. **The trial lens(es) should be placed:**
   a) With the sphere closest to the eye, and as close to the eye as possible
   b) With the cylinder closest to the eye, and as close to the eye as possible
   c) With the sphere closest to the eye at the patient's habitual vertex distance
   d) With the cylinder closest to the eye at the patient's habitual vertex distance

145. **Your Goldmann visual field patient is a 65-year-old aphake with the following glasses prescription OD: +10.00 sphere, with a +3.00 add. You want to use a contact lens to map the outer isopters (beyond 30 degrees), then add a trial lens for the central fields. The contact lens power you should choose is:**
   a) +8.00 sph
   b) +10.00 sph
   c) +11.00 sph
   d) +15.00 sph

146. **The Roman numeral designations on the Goldmann filter levers refer to stimulus:**
   a) Brightness
   b) Grayness
   c) Size
   d) Speed

147. **Regarding the Arabic number and alphabetic levers on the Goldmann perimeter:**
   a) The Arabic numbers designate stimulus size and the alphabet designates stimulus intensity
   b) The Arabic numbers designate 0.5 log units and the alphabet designates 0.1 log units of diminished light transmission
   c) The Arabic numbers designate 0.1 log units and the alphabet designates 0.5 log units of diminished light transmission
   d) The Arabic numbers designate stimulus intensity and the alphabet designates duration of presentation

148. **In Goldmann perimetry, if the patient's vision is hand motion or finger counting, it makes the most sense first to try mapping the outermost isopter using which target?**
   a) I4e
   b) I2e
   c) V4e
   d) VI6f

149. **Before starting Goldmann or automated fields, it is a good idea to perform a confrontation field on the patient. In addition to providing the examiner general information about possible gross defects, this serves to:**
   a) Indicate a possible starting threshold setting
   b) Educate the patient about fixation and response
   c) Quantitate possible defects
   d) Evaluate the patient's visual acuity

150. **Occlusion of the eye not being tested on visual fields is best done with:**
    a) Any pirate patch that is comfortable
    b) The patient's hand
    c) A piece of tape running from upper to lower lid
    d) A white patch

151. **The visual field patient should be told all of the following *except*:**
    a) You won't see every light right away
    b) Some of the lights will be dimmer or smaller than others
    c) Be sure to look at the light once you see it
    d) Press the button as soon as you're aware of the light

152. **The visual field patient should be positioned so that she:**
    a) Is not leaning forward at all
    b) Is on an eye level with the fixation area
    c) Has her chin jutted forward as far as possible
    d) Has her forehead tilted forward as far as possible

153. **What is the best way for a visual field patient who is physically unable to push the buzzer button with the thumb to indicate his response?**
    a) The test cannot be done
    b) Have him push the upside down buzzer against his leg or table top
    c) Have him give a verbal response
    d) Have him nod when he sees the stimulus

154. **If the visual field patient's head is tucked into a chin-down position:**
    a) The brow may obstruct the upper field
    b) The cheek bone may obstruct the lower field
    c) The eye cannot be aligned properly
    d) Fixation will be impossible

155. **If a visual field patient has a beard:**
    a) Tape the facial hair back out of the way
    b) Request that he shave before the test
    c) Position him so there is as little hair as possible in the chin rest
    d) No special modifications are necessary

156. **Which of the following is more comfortable during the visual field exam?**
    a) The feet should not touch the floor
    b) The back should be curved gently
    c) The patient should not have to lean forward at all
    d) The back should be straight, with feet flat on floor

157. **Adaptations that might allow a wheelchair-bound patient to be positioned at the perimeter include all of the following *except*:**
    a) Placing a sturdy board across the wheelchair armrests and having the patient sit on the board
    b) Raising the table so the chair will fit under it, and using pillows to help prop the patient
    c) Removing the wheelchair armrests so that the chair will slide under the table
    d) Removing the footrests so the chair will fit closer to the table

158. **In general, the longer the test time:**
    a) The less reliable the patient becomes
    b) The more reproducible the test
    c) The more accurate the test because more data is provided
    d) The more reliable the patient becomes

159. **To provide for patient comfort and rest during an automated visual field, the patient should be:**
    a) Told to hold down the button to pause the test after every couple of stimuli
    b) Told to close his eye whenever needed
    c) Encouraged periodically to continue, then allowed to rest between testing eyes
    d) Allowed to take a break every 5 minutes

160. **The patient should be warned not to sit back suddenly during a Goldmann visual field test because:**
    a) This will make the test take longer
    b) This will interrupt fixation and invalidate the test
    c) It is difficult to realign the patient
    d) He might come into contact with the projector arm

161. **Once the visual field patient has been instructed and is positioned properly:**
    a) Map the blind spot to ensure fixation
    b) Determine threshold to find a starting place
    c) Begin testing immediately to reduce patient fatigue
    d) Show a few static stimuli to acquaint the patient with the procedure

162. **You are halfway through the field when your patient begins to complain that her eye is stinging and watering. This might indicate that you forgot to instruct the patient to:**
    a) Maintain fixation
    b) Use artificial tears before the test
    c) Blink often during the test
    d) Take her allergy medication before the test

163. **Once the automated visual field test has begun, the perimetrist should:**
    a) Encourage the patient frequently
    b) Be totally quiet
    c) Leave the room
    d) Speak only if the patient repeatedly loses fixation

164. **The automated screening test that evaluates only one isopter border and finds deep scotomas is:**
    a) Infrathreshold single stimulus
    b) Suprathreshold single stimulus
    c) Infrathreshold multiple stimulus
    d) Suprathreshold multiple stimulus

165. **The *least* accurate test to use in computerized perimetry of glaucoma is the:**
    a) Three-zone format
    b) Hill of vision profile
    c) Comprehensive threshold evaluation
    d) Single stimulus suprathreshold

166. **An automated perimetry test that evaluates points by showing a single stimulus that is slightly brighter than the expected norm is:**
    a) Hill of vision profile
    b) Two-zone format
    c) Three-zone format
    d) Bracketing

167. **Instead of merely giving a "seen or unseen" yes/no type of answer, the three-zone format in automated perimetry:**
    a) Gives threshold readings for every point tested
    b) Provides more critical information of Bjerrum's and other areas
    c) Gives a three-dimensional printout
    d) Determines if a scotoma is relative or absolute

168. **The "quantify defects" strategy in automated perimetry is like a three-zone format, *except* that:**
    a) The number of absolute defects is counted and compared to a standard
    b) The number of relative defects is counted and compared to a standard
    c) The threshold of points missed on the single-intensity screening is determined
    d) The threshold of all points tested is determined during screening

169. **A full-field suprathreshold test would be appropriate for:**
    a) The glaucoma suspect
    b) The patient with known glaucoma
    c) The patient with 2.0 mm pupils
    d) General screening

170. **When testing a return patient for an annual automated field exam, it is important to:**
    a) Use the same test parameters as the previous test
    b) Use the same correcting lens as before
    c) Not fatigue the patient with test instructions
    d) Save the results on the same floppy disk

171. **The most commonly used automated visual field programs test points that are:**
    a) 2 degrees apart
    b) 6 degrees apart
    c) 20 degrees apart
    d) 30 degrees apart

172. **In order to detect steps on the vertical or horizontal meridians, automated test arrays are chosen that:**
    a) Lie directly on the vertical and horizontal meridians
    b) Straddle the vertical and horizontal meridians by 6 degrees
    c) Straddle the vertical and horizontal meridians by 2 or 3 degrees
    d) Are more compressed centrally

173. **An automated array suited for glaucoma testing might not be appropriate in other optic nerve disease because:**
    a) The blind spot is not checked as thoroughly
    b) The central 30 degrees is not checked as thoroughly
    c) The array designed for glaucoma may de-emphasize temporal points
    d) The array designed for glaucoma may de-emphasize nasal points

174. **If a defect includes or is close to fixation, it would be best to choose an automated test array that:**
    a) Checks points that are 2 degrees apart for the entire field
    b) Checks points that are 2 degrees apart in the central 10 degrees
    c) Provides a wider variety of stimuli
    d) Utilizes a red test object

175. **Which of the following automated threshold strategies would be most appropriate for a patient with optic neuritis?**
    a) Using results of a previous test
    b) Determining threshold at a point in each quadrant
    c) Full-field at 2 dB more intense than a previous test
    d) Using age-related normals

176. **Your physician-employer has sent a patient to you for automated full threshold visual field testing. Five minutes into the test it is obvious that the patient is physically unable to cope with threshold testing. You should:**
    a) Increase stimulus size
    b) Switch to a screening strategy
    c) Stop the test and inform the physician it is impossible
    d) Stop the test and re-educate the patient

177. **Fixation losses may be minimized by:**
    a) Telling the patient where the next kinetic stimulus is going to come from
    b) Telling the patient that you can see his eye during testing
    c) Use of the correct near add
    d) Enlarging the fixation point for every patient

178. **Match the automated field terms with the definitions. Some may be used more than once.**

    Terms:
    A. Fixation loss
    B. False positive
    C False negative
    D. Fluctuation

    Definitions:
    a) Evaluates the patient's understanding of the test
    b) The patient does not respond to the brightest target available in an area where he previously responded to a dimmer light
    c) The patient responds to a target that appears within the previously designated blind spot
    d) The patient responds to the sound of the perimeter when no stimulus was presented
    e) A measure of the patient's consistency
    f) Evaluates the patient's alertness
    g) Some perimeters will retest the points that were evaluated just before this occurred
    h) This factor can be affected by certain eye diseases
    i) A higher number indicates that the patient is giving varying responses to the same point
    j) May be detected continually by a photoelectric sensor

179. **During automated visual fields, if the patient repeatedly responds to the blind spot check, yet seems to be maintaining fixation:**
    a) Encourage the patient to continue to fixate
    b) Relocate the blind spot or reduce the fixation stimulus
    c) Pause the test and allow the patient to rest
    d) Turn off the fixation check

180. **In automated instruments that use an infrared monitor to evaluate fixation:**
    a) A fixation loss in a patient with blue eyes will register more easily than in a patient with brown eyes
    b) A fixation loss in a patient with brown eyes will register more easily than in a patient with blue eyes
    c) Having the patient wear a soft contact lens will increase the sensitivity of the monitor
    d) A correcting lens cannot be used because it will interfere with the monitor

181. **The term "catch trials" refers to:**
    a) Methods used in automated perimetry to ensure reproducible fields
    b) Methods used in manual/Goldmann perimetry to ensure reliable fields
    c) Methods used in automated perimetry to rate patient reliability
    d) The trial lens used during the central part of a field test

182. **Common errors in testing the central 30 degrees include all of the following *except*:**
    a) Forgetting to remove the correcting lens
    b) Presenting static targets in a steady rhythm
    c) Using a stimulus that stretches the isopter beyond 30 degrees
    d) Moving the stimulus too quickly, creating a falsely enlarged blind spot

183. **A field with artificially contracted isopters and a larger than normal blind spot could be caused by:**
    a) A test stimulus that is too large or bright
    b) Slow response time on the part of the patient
    c) Moving the stimulus too slowly
    d) Oscillating the stimulus

184. **The most common areas for artifacts in the visual field are:**
    a) Superior nasal or inferior nasal
    b) Superior temporal or inferior temporal
    c) Temporal nasal or superior nasal
    d) Nasal temporal or inferior temporal

185. **The chances of producing a correcting lens artifact on visual field testing can be reduced by:**
    a) Using only wide-rimmed trial lenses
    b) Using spherical correction and placing it as close to the eye as possible
    c) Using the proper lens and placing it as close to the eye as possible
    d) Using the proper lens to test the field beyond the central 30 degrees

186. **Selecting a correcting lens of improper power may result in:**
    a) Apparent field depression
    b) Artificial enlargement of the blind spot
    c) Misplacement of the blind spot
    d) Spiral fields

187. **Match the following visual fields to the artifacts (Figures 4-3 through 4-6):**
    Ptotic upper eyelid
    Thick rim on correcting lens
    Hysteria or malingering
    Decentered correcting lens
    a) Figure 4-3
    b) Figure 4-4
    c) Figure 4-5
    d) Figure 4-6

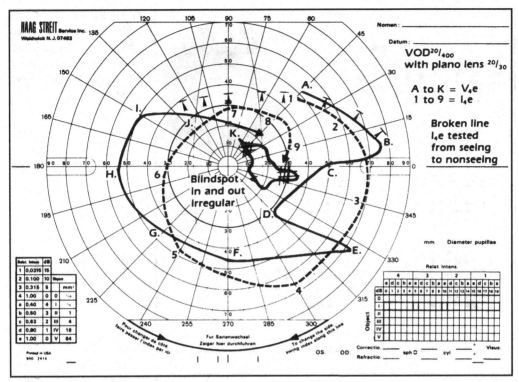

a) **Figure 4-3.** Reprinted with permission from Garber N. *Visual Field Examination*. Thorofare, NJ: SLACK Incorporated; 1998.

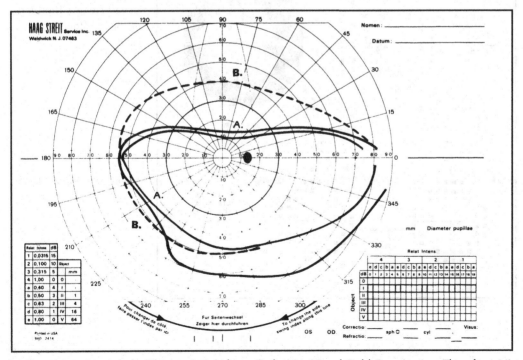

b) **Figure 4-4.** Reprinted with permission from Garber N. *Visual Field Examination*. Thorofare, NJ: SLACK Incorporated; 1998.

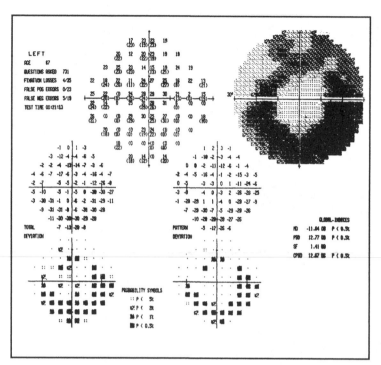

c) **Figure 4-5.** Reprinted with permission from Choplin N, Edwards R. *Visual Fields*. Thorofare, NJ: SLACK Incorporated; 1998.

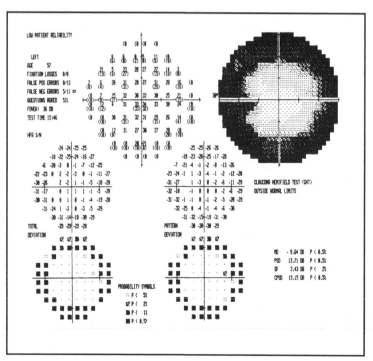

d) **Figure 4-6.** Reprinted with permission from Choplin N, Edwards R. *Visual Fields*. Thorofare, NJ: SLACK Incorporated; 1998.

188. **All of the following are characteristics of retinal area defects** *except*:
    a) Defects at this level are binocular
    b) Most field-related pathology also is visible with the ophthalmoscope
    c) They can cross the vertical and horizontal meridians
    d) Defects are projected into the opposite quadrant

189. **If a retinal detachment is found in the superior nasal retina, where is the corresponding field loss?**
    a) Superior nasal
    b) Superior temporal
    c) Inferior nasal
    d) Inferior temporal

190. **The retinal field defect that results in the most visual limitation occurs in the:**
    a) Bjerrum fibers
    b) Periphery
    c) Macula
    d) Disc

191. **Damage in the nerve fiber layer commonly produces which of the following field defects?**
    a) Hemianopsias
    b) Quadrantanopsias
    c) Congruous
    d) Bjerrum scotomas

192. **In the case where nerve fiber layer damage has caused a constriction in the isopter, the isopter will:**
    a) Progress toward the horizontal meridian
    b) Progress toward the disc
    c) Progress toward the vertical meridian
    d) Show no particular pattern of progression

193. **Common characteristics of nerve fiber layer defects include all of the following** *except*:
    a) Arc-shaped constrictions or contractions
    b) Nasal step
    c) Enlarged blind spot
    d) Left homonymous hemianopsia

194. **Which of the following has no resulting field loss?**
    a) Optic neuritis
    b) Macular hole
    c) Ocular hypertension
    d) Central retinal artery occlusion

195. **Enlargement of the blind spot might typically be expected to occur in all of the following conditions** *except*:
    a) Glaucoma
    b) Retinal detachment
    c) Papilledema (papillitis)
    d) Optic nerve coloboma

196. **Except in glaucoma, enlargement of the blind spot caused by optic nerve damage generally is:**
    a) Oriented vertically
    b) Oriented horizontally
    c) Rounded or concentric
    d) Tapered at the top

197. **The most common visual field defect found in optic nerve damage is:**
    a) Nasal step
    b) Enlarged blind spot
    c) Central scotoma
    d) Bjerrum's scotoma

198. **Optic nerve damage that causes a visual field defect in both eyes cannot occur anterior to:**
    a) The junction of the optic nerve and the chiasm
    b) The chiasm
    c) Where the fibers leave the chiasm
    d) The optic tract

199. **All of the following regarding field loss in optic neuritis are true *except*:**
    a) Field loss is permanent
    b) The most common defect is a central scotoma
    c) It can cause a defect anywhere in the nerve fiber bundle
    d) Centrocecal defects can also occur

200. **Optic disc drusen can cause field defects that mimic:**
    a) Retinal detachment
    b) Glaucoma
    c) Pituitary tumor
    d) Hysteria

201. **The most common field defect in optic disc drusen is:**
    a) Progressive contractions
    b) Localized depressions
    c) Scotomas
    d) Inferior nasal step

202. **A patient taking Plaquenil (hydroxychloroquine) should have periodic visual field examinations to check for:**
    a) Bitemporal hemianopsia
    b) Temporal wedge
    c) Nasal step
    d) Paracentral scotoma

203. **Which areas are most important when screening for glaucomatous defects?**
    a) Fovea, superior, and temporal
    b) Central 30 degrees
    c) Outer 30 degrees
    d) Nasal, central 20 degrees, and blind spot

204. **The standard perimetric screening technique for detecting glaucomatous defects is:**
    a) Armaly/Drance
    b) Goldmann
    c) Overlapping fields
    d) Hesse

205. **Changes in the visual field of the glaucoma patient correspond to:**
    a) IOP readings
    b) Choroidal blood supply to the retina
    c) The progression of nerve fiber bundle damage at the rim of the optic disc
    d) How far posteriorly into the visual pathway the damage has progressed

206. **The nasal contraction seen in the glaucomatous field is:**
    a) An inferior nasal step
    b) A superior nasal step
    c) A vertical nasal step
    d) Attached to the blind spot

207. **The most common initial field loss(es) seen in open-angle glaucoma is/are:**
    a) Central scotoma and vertical step
    b) Nasal step
    c) Paracentral scotoma and nasal step
    d) Temporal wedge and arcuate scotoma

208. **The Bjerrum scotomas seen in open-angle glaucoma occur in which eccentricity?**
    a) 7.5 degrees
    b) 15 degrees
    c) 30 degrees
    d) 45 degrees

209. **The very last area of the visual field remaining in end-stage glaucoma is the:**
    a) Nasal step
    b) Blind spot
    c) Central 5 degrees
    d) Temporal crescent

210. **In general, the more congruous the defect, the more likely that the problem site is:**
    a) Prechiasmal
    b) Related to the optic nerve
    c) More posteriorly located
    d) More anteriorly located

211. **One hallmark of the neurological field is:**
    a) Respect for the vertical meridian
    b) Respect for the horizontal meridian
    c) The macula is never affected
    d) The blind spot is never affected

212. **Which location should be screened when ruling out a neurological defect?**
    a) The horizontal meridian
    b) The vertical meridian
    c) The central 20 degrees
    d) The nasal area

213. **A total homonymous hemianopsia can occur in all of the following *except*:**
    a) The optic nerve
    b) The optic tract
    c) The temporal lobe
    d) The occipital lobe

214. **Bitemporal field defects can occur *only* in the:**
    a) Retina
    b) Optic nerve
    c) Chiasm
    d) Temporal lobe

215. **"Pie-in-the-sky" and "pie-on-the-floor" defects are indications of damage in the:**
    a) Optic tract
    b) Lateral geniculate body
    c) Optic radiations
    d) Visual cortex

216. **Scintillating (shimmering or flickering) scotomas are sometimes seen in:**
    a) Optic neuritis
    b) Angle-closure glaucoma
    c) Migraines
    d) Retinitis pigmentosa

217. **Field patterns typical of a hysterical patient include all of the following *except*:**
    a) Spiral
    b) Star-shaped
    c) Tubular
    d) Square

218. **Hysterical visual field loss is usually a product of:**
    a) The patient's desire to fool the examiner
    b) Elevated IOP
    c) Mental conflict
    d) Pseudotumor cerebri

219. **Which technique is more useful in determining nonorganic visual field loss?**
    a) Automated full-field threshold
    b) Confrontation fields
    c) Amsler grid
    d) Goldmann fields

220. **In automated testing, one clue that field loss may be nonfunctional is:**
    a) A field loss pattern that is not later reproduced
    b) High rate of fixation loss
    c) Presence of gray scale artifacts
    d) Generalized constriction

221. **All of the following findings commonly occur in nonfunctional field loss as exhibited on automated fields *except*:**
    a) Severe constriction
    b) Enlarged blind spot
    c) Normal foveal threshold levels
    d) Decreased visual acuity

222. Match the visual field to the most likely diagnosis (Figures 4-7 through 4-13):

Diagnosis:

Chiasmal defect

Glaucoma

Nerve fiber layer defect

Nonorganic defect

Optic disc drusen

Postchiasmal defect

Retinal detachment

a) Figure 4-7

b) Figure 4-8

c) Figure 4-9

d) Figure 4-10

e) Figure 4-11

f) Figure 4-12

g) Figure 4-13

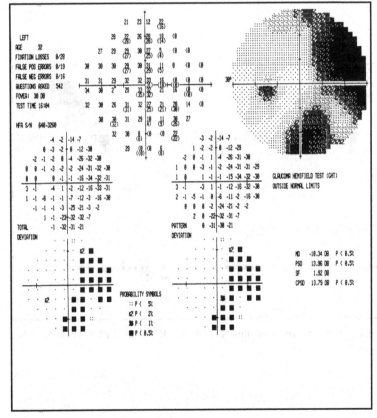

a) **Figure 4-7.** Reprinted with permission from Choplin N, Edwards R. *Visual Fields*. Thorofare, NJ: SLACK Incorporated; 1998.

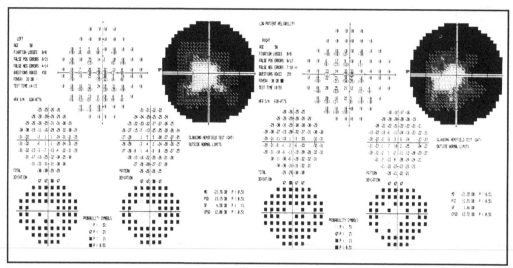

b) Figure 4-8. Reprinted with permission from Choplin N, Edwards R. *Visual Fields*. Thorofare, NJ: SLACK Incorporated; 1998.

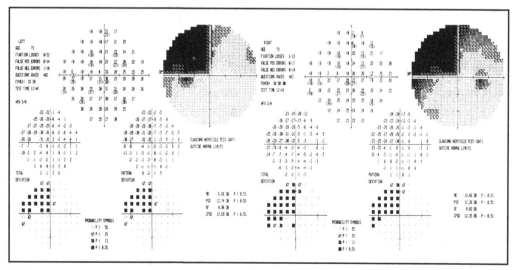

c) Figure 4-9. Reprinted with permission from Choplin N, Edwards R. *Visual Fields*. Thorofare, NJ: SLACK Incorporated; 1998.

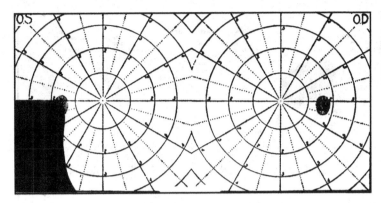

d) **Figure 4-10.** Reprinted with permission from Garber N. *Visual Field Examination*. Thorofare, NJ: SLACK Incorporated; 1998.

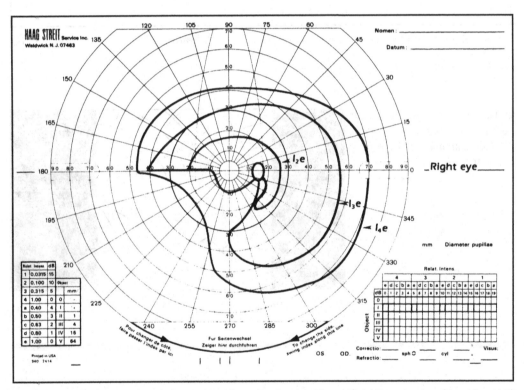

e) **Figure 4-11.** Reprinted with permission from Garber N. *Visual Field Examination*. Thorofare, NJ: SLACK Incorporated; 1998.

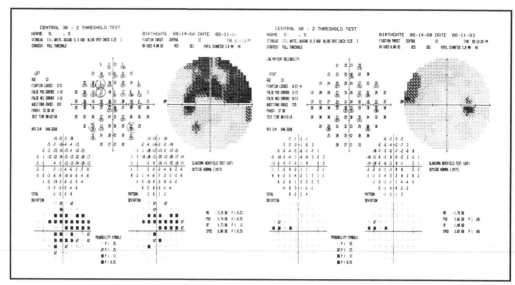

f) Figure 4-12. Reprinted with permission from Choplin N, Edwards R. *Visual Fields*. Thorofare, NJ: SLACK Incorporated; 1998.

g) Figure 4-13. Reprinted with permission from Garber N. *Visual Field Examination*. Thorofare, NJ: SLACK Incorporated; 1998.

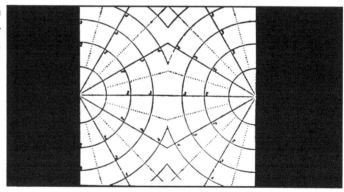

Chapter 5

Contact Lenses

1. **Most practitioners would prefer to fit a gas permeable lens instead of a traditional hard (PMMA) lens because:**
   a) Vision with a gas permeable lens is better
   b) Gas permeable lenses are easier to handle
   c) Gas permeable lenses are available for astigmatism
   d) Corneal warpage is less with gas permeable lenses

2. **In spite of the current popularity of gas permeable and soft lenses, PMMA lenses are still useful in cases of:**
   a) High astigmatism
   b) High hyperopia
   c) High myopia
   d) Presbyopia

3. **A PMMA lens would be contraindicated in all of the following *except*:**
   a) Ectatic corneal dystrophy
   b) Corneal anesthesia
   c) Lid anomalies
   d) Dry eye

4. **The characteristics of PMMA material include all of the following *except*:**
   a) Resists warpage
   b) Oxygen permeable
   c) Wets well
   d) Easy to clean

5. **Because of the characteristics of PMMA lenses, almost all PMMA lens wearers have some degree of:**
   a) Injection
   b) Photophobia
   c) Corneal anoxia
   d) Neovascularization

6. **The characteristic of soft lens material that is responsible for most of the lens's advantages (and disadvantages) is its:**
   a) Tear exchange under the lens
   b) Ability to absorb water
   c) Resistance to deposits
   d) Larger diameter

7. **Soft lens material includes all of the following polymers *except*:**
   a) Hydrogel
   b) Silicone
   c) CAB (cellulose acetate butyrate)
   d) HEMA (hydroxyethylmethacrylate)

8. **The lower the water content of a soft lens:**
   a) The more durable the lens
   b) The greater oxygen permeability
   c) The less frequently it needs to be cleaned
   d) The smaller the diameter

9. **The advantages of soft lenses include all of the following *except*:**
   a) They are more comfortable than rigid lenses
   b) They provide crisper vision than rigid lenses
   c) They can be worn intermittently
   d) There is less lens loss

10. **Which patient is a poor candidate for soft lenses?**
    a) A patient with dry eye
    b) A patient with a spherical refractive error
    c) An infant or child
    d) A recreational basketball player

11. **One of the main disadvantages to soft lenses is:**
    a) Frequent lens loss
    b) Poor durability
    c) Low oxygen permeability
    d) Corneal injury on insertion

12. **One of the main risks of wearing soft contact lenses is:**
    a) Modifications are impossible
    b) Residual astigmatism
    c) Infection
    d) Lens discoloration

13. **All of the following are contraindications to soft toric lenses *except*:**
    a) Lenticular astigmatism
    b) Irregular corneal astigmatism
    c) Inadequate lid closure
    d) Impaired blink reflex

14. **The major difficulty with fitting toric lenses is:**
    a) Patient discomfort
    b) Lens stability on the eye
    c) Arriving at the correct prescription
    d) Obtaining accurate over-refractions

15. **Matching. Match the toric lens stabilization method with its definition.**

Terms:	Definitions:
A. Aspheric back surface	a) Weights the bottom part of the lens with prism
B. Bioflange	b) A flat edge on the bottom portion of the lens
C. Dynamic stabilization	c) A thin edge on the top and bottom portions of the lens with a thicker center
D. Posterior toric	d) Toric correction is on the back of the lens, where it can physically "match up" to the cornea
E. Prism ballast	e) Creates drag between the lens edge and the periphery of the cornea
F. Truncation	f) Weights the lens with a thick bottom edge

16. **A soft toric lens that is thick across the belly and thinned-out at the top and bottom is called a:**
    a) Double slab-off lens
    b) Prism ballast lens
    c) Bi-toric lens
    d) Truncated lens

17. **An aid in evaluating the stability of a soft toric lens is:**
    a) The movement gauge
    b) Etch or laser marks on the lens
    c) A protractor in the slit lamp ocular
    d) The contact lens gauge

18. **An easy method to remember how to compensate for an off-axis soft toric lens is:**
    a) SAM/FAP
    b) LARS
    c) TAM
    d) Roy G. Biv

19. **If lens rotation is to the left, one should add the number of degrees of rotation to the:**
    a) Axis of the contact lens
    b) Axis of the steepest K reading
    c) Axis of the flattest K reading
    d) Axis of the patient's refraction

20. **The major factor(s) influencing toric soft lens stability is/are:**
    a) The weighting and truncating of the lens
    b) The contour, position, and tightness of the lids
    c) The patient's K readings
    d) The thickness and water content of the lens polymer

21. **Toric rigid lenses may be required by patients:**
    a) Whose refractive and corneal astigmatism agree in power but not in axis
    b) With spherical corneas and lenticular astigmatism
    c) Whose corneal astigmatism is greater than their refractive astigmatism
    d) All of the above

22. **Decentration and rocking of a gas permeable lens caused by astigmatism may be compensated for by using a:**
    a) Larger lens
    b) Smaller lens
    c) Piggyback system
    d) Higher power lens

23. **A patient with a highly toric cornea may require a gas permeable lens that is:**
    a) Thinner or more flexible
    b) Thicker or more rigid
    c) Higher in water content
    d) Thicker at the edges

24. **The amount of astigmatism that is present after the patient is fitted with lenses is referred to as:**
    a) Residual astigmatism
    b) Corneal astigmatism
    c) Lenticular astigmatism
    d) Irregular astigmatism

25. **The most common cause of residual astigmatism in contact lens wearers is:**
    a) The tear lens
    b) The cornea
    c) The crystalline lens
    d) The retina

26. **With spherical soft lenses, a small amount of corneal astigmatism is:**
    a) Masked
    b) Eliminated
    c) Tolerated
    d) A reason to fit toric lenses

27. **The patient with astigmatism may tolerate spherical soft contact lenses up to the point that the astigmatism is:**
    a) Less than 1/3 of the total refractive error
    b) Less that 1/2 of the total refractive error
    c) Lenticular
    d) With the rule

28. **The patient with astigmatism may tolerate a spherical rigid contact lens if the astigmatism is:**
    a) With the rule
    b) Against the rule
    c) 3.00 diopters or more
    d) 3.00 diopters or less

29. **Simultaneous vision bifocal contact lenses:**
    a) Involve fitting one eye for distance and the other eye for near
    b) Are not available with progressive power
    c) Have a reading segment at the bottom of the lens
    d) Have distance correction in the center and near correction in an outer ring

30. **The limiting factor in fitting simultaneous bifocal contacts is:**
    a) The size of the patient's pupil
    b) The patient's K readings
    c) The patient's corneal diameter
    d) The patient's lid position

31. **The most common visual complaint with simultaneous bifocal contacts is:**
    a) Ghost images
    b) Loss of depth perception
    c) Loss of binocularity
    d) Inability to coordinate the eyes

32. **The reverse design simultaneous bifocal contact lenses involves:**
    a) Using the opposite eyes for distance and near
    b) Having the near segment at the top of the lens
    c) Having near correction in the center and the distance correction in the outer ring
    d) Wearing contacts for near and glasses to overcorrect at distance

33. **A patient with reverse simultaneous bifocal contact lenses will find that in very bright light, he:**
    a) Can only see at a distance
    b) Can only see up close
    c) Can only see with the right eye
    d) Must wear glasses

34. **Alternating vision bifocal contact lenses:**
    a) Are another term for monofit
    b) Have a bull's-eye for near in the center for one eye, and for distance in the other
    c) Can be fit for one eye only
    d) Have an upper segment for distance and a lower segment for near

35. **In addition to patient motivation, successful fit of alternating vision bifocal contact lenses depends on:**
    a) Whether the patient is right- or left-handed
    b) The position of the lower lid
    c) The patient's age
    d) The strength of add required

36. **If the patient is wearing alternating vision bifocal contact lenses and is attempting to read prices on a shelf above shoulder level:**
    a) The print will be clear
    b) The print will be blurred
    c) The lenses will rotate
    d) The lenses will move out of alignment

37. **An advantage of gas permeable bifocal contact lenses vs. soft bifocal contact lenses in an alternating vision design is:**
    a) Gas permeable lenses are more comfortable
    b) Gas permeable lenses are not as dependent on lid positioning
    c) It is easier for the patient to "find" the right spot to look through
    d) Most patients adapt to them easily

38. **Monovision contact lens fitting for presbyopia involves:**
    a) Fitting both eyes for distance and using reading glasses for near
    b) Fitting one eye (usually the dominant eye) for distance, and the other eye for near
    c) Fitting one eye (usually the dominant eye) for near, and the other eye for distance
    d) Wearing a contact lens for near in one eye and leaving the other eye uncorrected

39. **Which of the following probably would be a poor candidate for the monofit technique?**
    a) A public speaker
    b) A teacher
    c) A bookkeeper
    d) An actor

40. **Patients using the monovision technique might experience problems:**
    a) Taking the driver's license vision test
    b) In very bright light
    c) Looking from the desk to the board in classroom situations
    d) When their peripheral vision is checked by confrontation

41. **Fewer and fewer patients are needing aphakic contact lens correction because:**
    a) Aphakic glasses have improved
    b) Contact lenses are difficult for older patients to handle
    c) Contact lenses are difficult for aphakic patients to see
    d) Intraocular lenses (IOLs) are highly successful

42. **Considerations for fitting contacts on the average aphakic eye include all of the following *except*:**
    a) Dryness
    b) Senility
    c) Lid laxity
    d) Tendency for superior neovascularization

43. **When an aphakic patient switches from glasses to contact lenses, objects will appear to be:**
    a) Closer
    b) Farther away
    c) More brightly colored
    d) Less distinct

44. **When teaching an aphakic patient to handle soft contact lenses, it is important to remember that he:**
    a) Also will need a caregiver trained in lens handling
    b) Cannot see the lenses when the glasses are off
    c) Has no corneal sensation and cannot tell when the lens is on
    d) Must be taught to use a plunger for lens removal

45. **In order to reduce the weight of a high plus lens and to improve centration, rigid contact lenses for aphakia should be:**
    a) Fenestrated
    b) Truncated
    c) Lenticularized
    d) Prism ballasted

46. **In the design referred to above, the lens power is ground:**
    a) On the bowl
    b) On the carrier
    c) Above the flattened edge
    d) Above the prism

47. **In the design referred to above, a high plus lens will incorporate:**
    a) A hyperprism
    b) A myoprism
    c) A hyperflange
    d) A myoflange

48. **The thick edge of the rigid aphakic lens design referred to above:**
    a) Weighs the contact down
    b) Prevents lens movement
    c) Is held up by the upper lid
    d) Rests on the lower lid margin

49. **If the patient had phacoemulsification with a small incision, a soft contact lens may often be fitted:**
    a) 24 hours after surgery
    b) 1 week after surgery
    c) 1 month after surgery
    d) 4 months after surgery

50. **If a soft contact lens is fitted on an aphake too soon after surgery while corneal edema is still present, 1 day's wear may cause:**
    a) A loss of endothelial cells
    b) A loss of epithelial cells
    c) Corneal neovascularization
    d) Conjunctival injection

51. **In order to stabilize the heavier high plus soft contact lens used in aphakia:**
    a) The lens is fenestrated
    b) The corneal apex should be vaulted
    c) A smaller diameter is used
    d) A larger diameter is used

52. **All of the following are poor candidates for extended wear lenses *except*:**
    a) Those who work in a dusty environment
    b) Those with chronic blepharitis
    c) Those taking blood thinners
    d) Those with pre-existing giant papillary conjunctivitis (GPC)

53. **A patient with decreased tearing who is fit with high water content extended wear soft lenses may notice that:**
    a) A smaller diameter is more comfortable
    b) Deposits form at an increased rate
    c) The lenses move excessively
    d) Tear production improves

54. **One disadvantage of a low water content extended wear soft lens is:**
    a) Low resistance to heat
    b) Low resistance to deposits
    c) Responds erratically to environmental changes
    d) Little lens movement

55. **Which of the following statements regarding extended wear is most accurate?**
    a) High water content extended wear lenses are both heat and deposit resistant
    b) Low water content lenses may respond erratically to environmental changes
    c) The current trend is to discourage long-term extended wear
    d) Neovascularization rarely occurs in aphakes

56. **Patients who remove their extended wear lenses only once a month experience a higher percentage of all of the following *except*:**
    a) Decreased need for artificial lubrication
    b) Redness
    c) Corneal anesthesia
    d) Exposure keratitis when lenses are removed

57. **Every patient who wears extended wear contact lenses should be told to:**
    a) Remove the lenses and clean them daily
    b) Allow the lenses to remain in the eye for up to 1 month
    c) Use lubricating drops every morning and during the day
    d) Endure occasional pain and redness as a matter of course

58. **"Myopic creep" is a gradual increase in myopia that sometimes occurs in extended wear. It is caused by:**
    a) Corneal edema
    b) Neovascularization
    c) Microcyst formation
    d) Injection

59. **Extended wear soft lenses should generally be replaced:**
    a) Every month
    b) Every 3 to 6 months
    c) Annually
    d) Only when ruined by deposits

60. **Disadvantages of rigid GP extended wear lenses include all of the following *except*:**
    a) Increased incidence of neovascularization
    b) Adhering of the lens overnight
    c) Lens displacement during sleep
    d) Corneal distortion

61. **The aphakic cornea can tolerate a +12.00 extended wear contact lens better than a phakic eye because:**
    a) The lens can be fenestrated
    b) An aphake has less corneal sensation
    c) The patients usually are highly motivated
    d) An aphakic eye requires less oxygen

62. **A good general rule for fitting extended wear lenses is to:**
    a) Fit the highest water content possible
    b) Fit the loosest lens possible
    c) Fit gas permeable whenever possible
    d) Fit the smallest diameter possible

63. **The fact that gas permeable material allows more oxygen to the eye means that:**
    a) The lens can be larger than a PMMA lens
    b) The lens is more comfortable than a PMMA lens
    c) Lens movement is not an important factor
    d) The lens can be allowed to rest on the lower lid margin

64. **The average life of a rigid gas permeable lens is:**
    a) 6 to 9 months
    b) 12 months
    c) 18 to 24 months
    d) 36 months

65. **A disadvantage of the higher Dk value gas permeable lenses is:**
    a) Excessive movement
    b) Excessive thickness
    c) A smaller lens must be used
    d) Increased tendency to warp

66. **Which of the following makes a patient a poor candidate for gas permeable contact lenses?**
    a) History of GPC
    b) Exophthalmos
    c) Corneal irregularity
    d) Neovascularization from soft lenses

67. **All of the following are gas permeable contact lens materials *except*:**
    a) Hydroxyethyl methacrylate (HEMA)
    b) CAB
    c) Silicone/acrylate
    d) Fluoropolymers

68. **Which of the following is *not* a shortcoming of high silicone content gas permeable contact lenses?**
    a) Wets poorly
    b) Decreased Dk value
    c) Increased deposit formation
    d) Lens chipping and cracking

69. **Current fitting philosophy for gas permeable lenses dictates that:**
    a) The upper lid should control lens movement
    b) The lens should rest on the lower lid
    c) There should be as little movement as possible
    d) The lens should float down below the upper lid after each blink

70. **Advantages of the gas permeable lens include all of the following *except*:**
    a) Reduced spectacle blur
    b) No deposit formation
    c) Better centration
    d) Adaptation to full time wear in about 1 week

71. **Truncation is a method used to:**
    a) Increase comfort of a toric lens
    b) Increase oxygen supply to the cornea
    c) Provide stability to a toric lens
    d) Decrease corneal dehydration

72. **In order to be most effective, truncation is best combined with:**
    a) Prism ballast
    b) Fenestration
    c) Glasses for overcorrection
    d) A piggyback lens system

73. **Problems that may occur in truncation of a single vision toric lens include all of the following *except*:**
    a) Difficulty with near vision
    b) A constant awareness of the lens edge
    c) Inferior corneal staining and injection
    d) Superior corneal dehydration and exposure

74. **In addition to astigmatism, truncated lenses also are used in the treatment of:**
    a) Dry eye
    b) Presbyopia
    c) Keratoconus
    d) Aphakia

75. **Bandage contact lenses are routinely used for all of the following *except*:**
    a) Correction of a refractive error
    b) Promoting healing and protection
    c) Patient comfort
    d) Drug reservoir

76. **The key in selecting a bandage contact lens is:**
    a) The patient's refractive error
    b) The patient's ability to handle the lens
    c) Oxygen permeability
    d) The patient's corneal curvature

77. **Even if a patient has a refractive error, it is best to try a plano bandage lens first because:**
    a) Refractive correction may trigger ciliary spasms
    b) A plano lens is thinner
    c) A plano lens has a higher water content
    d) The patient should avoid using the eye anyway

78. **All of the following are suitable bandage contact lenses *except*:**
    a) A collagen disintegrating lens
    b) A disposable soft lens
    c) A low water content lens
    d) A thin soft lens

79. **All of the following might be expected to be candidates for a bandage contact lens *except*:**
    a) Postoperative excimer laser treatment
    b) Recurrent corneal erosion syndrome
    c) Corneal ulcer
    d) No-stitch cataract extraction

80. **A rigid lens would *not* be a good choice for a drug reservoir because:**
    a) It is not as absorbent as a soft lens
    b) It does not provide as smooth a surface as a soft lens
    c) Its movement might irritate the cornea further
    d) It does not disintegrate like a soft lens

81. **If the injured corneal surface is *not* intact, then the bandage lens should be fit so that there is:**
    a) Normal movement
    b) Minimal or no movement
    c) No oxygen permeability
    d) Limbal exposure

82. **A patient with a bandage lens for a corneal abrasion or erosion should be advised that:**
    a) Discomfort may continue for the first day or two
    b) He needs to remove the lens at night
    c) He may use topical anesthetic as needed for comfort
    d) Increased comfort will be instantaneous

83. **The laboratory measurement of the oxygen permeability of a given material is the:**
    a) Water content
    b) Wetting angle
    c) Dk value
    d) Lens permeability coefficient

84. **The actual amount of oxygen that gets through the contact lens and reaches the cornea is a product of:**
    a) Lens material and design, and central and edge thickness
    b) The cylinder axis and movement on blinking
    c) A Schirmer's tear test and the water content of the lens
    d) Wearing time, lens solutions, and patient compliance

85. **The PMMA rigid lens essentially has no permeability. How does oxygen reach the cornea in PMMA lens wearers?**
    a) Through the eyelids
    b) Through the tears
    c) Through the choroidal blood vessels
    d) Through the conjunctiva

86. **The oxygen supply to the cornea can be increased by selecting a lens:**
    a) With a high Dk value or reduced thickness
    b) With a low Dk value or reduced thickness
    c) With a high Dk value or increased thickness
    d) With a low Dk value or increased thickness

87. **Corneal edema will occur if oxygen availability falls below:**
    a) 1.5 to 2.5%
    b) 7 to 10%
    c) 20%
    d) 30%

88. **Which of the following lenses has the highest oxygen permeability (Dk)?**
    a) PMMA
    b) HEMA
    c) CAB
    d) Silicone

89. **Radius can be defined as:**
    a) The distance around a sphere
    b) The distance from the center of a sphere to its edge
    c) The distance from one edge of a sphere to the other through the sphere's center
    d) The distance from the center of one sphere to another

90. **An understanding of the base curve of a contact lens can be visualized by thinking of the lens as:**
    a) A slice of a sphere
    b) A circle
    c) A slice of a cylinder
    d) A section of an ellipse

91. **The longer the radius of curvature of a contact lens:**
    a) The steeper the lens
    b) The flatter the lens
    c) The larger the diameter
    d) The greater the vault

92. **If you place a contact lens on a flat surface, the distance from the center of the lens to the flat surface would be a measurement of the lens's:**
    a) Base curve
    b) Diameter
    c) Vault
    d) Radius

93. **Which of the following statements regarding lens vault is *not* true?**
    a) The average patient should be fit with the highest vault possible
    b) A lens with a steeper vault will fit tighter
    c) Increasing lens diameter will steepen the vault
    d) Lengthening the radius of curvature will flatten the vault

94. **A line through the center of the contact lens from one edge to the other would be a measure of the lens's:**
    a) Sagittal depth
    b) Radius
    c) Base curve
    d) Diameter

95. **Increasing the diameter of a lens acts to:**
    a) Loosen the lens
    b) Tighten the lens
    c) Improve vision
    d) Increase oxygen transmission

96. **A common problem associated with thicker (higher power) contact lenses is:**
    a) Poor durability
    b) Poor optical quality
    c) Hypoxia
    d) Conjunctival drag

97. **A soft contact lens with a high water content will:**
    a) Be more stable if lens dehydration occurs
    b) Allow for greater oxygen transmission
    c) Need to be disinfected by thermal methods only
    d) Be more durable if it is made of HEMA

98. **The base curve of a rigid lens is found on:**
    a) The central posterior curve
    b) The intermediate curve
    c) The peripheral curve
    d) All curves

99. **The power of a rigid lens is ground on:**
    a) The optical zone
    b) The junctions
    c) The limbal zone
    d) The entire lens

100. **The smoothness or roughness of the junctions between adjacent curves on a rigid contact lens is referred to as:**
    a) Bevel
    b) Edging
    c) Lenticulation
    d) Blend

101. **In order to improve centration of a high minus lens, the edges might be tapered in a process known as:**
    a) Edging
    b) Fenestration
    c) Truncation
    d) Beveling

102. **In addition to the refractive error and residual astigmatism, when selecting the power for rigid contact lenses, one must also consider the:**
    a) Axial length
    b) Tear film
    c) Size of the fovea
    d) Endothelial cell count

103. **The keratometer:**
    a) Helps us to monitor changes in corneal curvature at the apex and in the periphery
    b) Is the only way to accurately measure the cornea of a patient with keratoconus
    c) Enables the user to view microscopic defects on a rigid lens
    d) Can be used to identify corneal warpage and rigid lens edema

104. **Number the following steps of using a keratometer in chronological order:**
    ___Occlude the eye not being tested
    ___Turn the drum so that the plus signs are aligned exactly tip-to-tip
    ___Turn the dials to superimpose the plus and minus signs
    ___Position the patient
    ___Focus the mires and center the cross hairs in the lower right hand circle
    ___Focus the eyepiece

105. **You are attempting a K reading and don't see both plus signs. This might be due to:**
    a) A drooped upper lid
    b) The patient closing his eye
    c) A keratometer occluder in the way
    d) Improper focusing

106. **Matching. Select one best answer.**

Probable condition:	Keratometer mires appear:
Flat cornea	a) Small
Corneal warpage	b) Round
Keratoconus	c) Elliptical
Spherical cornea	d) Very large
Steep cornea	e) Clear, then quickly blur
Dry eye	f) Wavy, blurred, discontinuous
Astigmatism	g) Distorted, small, can't superimpose

107. **If the cross hairs of the keratometer are *not* centered during the initial reading for contact lens fitting:**
    a) You may select a lens that is too strong
    b) The resulting fit may be too tight
    c) The resulting fit may be too loose
    d) You may select a lens that is too small

108. **Fitting soft lenses steeper than K usually will result in:**
    a) Good lens movement
    b) A minus tear layer under the lens
    c) Fluctuations in vision following the blink
    d) Excellent comfort and visual acuity

109. **Your patient has been wearing a soft lens for about 20 to 30 minutes. With the lenses still in place, you view the eye through the keratometer. The mires are blurred initially, but clear after a blink. This probably indicates:**
    a) The lens is too tight, too large, or too steep
    b) The lens is too loose, too small, or too flat
    c) The lens is "sucked on"
    d) The lens power is not adequate

110. **You have removed the patient's contacts and are evaluating the corneas with the keratometer. You note that the K readings are steeper than at the last visit, several months ago. This could indicate:**
    a) Corneal neovascularization
    b) Mechanical molding of the cornea
    c) Corneal edema
    d) Corneal ulcer

111. **If progressive corneal flattening or steepening occurs over a period of time in a contact lens wearer:**
    a) The patient should discontinue lens wear permanently
    b) You should adjust the power of the lens accordingly
    c) The cleaning solutions should be changed
    d) You should change lens material and/or design

112. **You want to fit a rigid contact lens, and the patient's K reading is 43.50/44.75. What base curve will you select to fit the patient "on K"?**
    a) 43.50
    b) 44.12
    c) 44.25
    d) 44.75

113. **For most contact lens fitting purposes, it is acceptable to measure corneal diameter:**
    a) Using an ophthalmoscope set on +10.0 and a millimeter rule
    b) By measuring the visible iris with a millimeter rule
    c) By using a pachymeter
    d) By anesthetizing the eye and using calipers

114. **The general rule about corneal diameter is:**
    a) Neither a rigid nor a soft lens should touch the limbus
    b) A soft lens should cover the cornea to the limbus, but not beyond
    c) The diameter of a rigid lens should exceed the corneal diameter by 1 mm
    d) Corneal diameter does not figure into the fit of any contact lens

115. **Patients with large pupils who are being fit for rigid lenses will require:**
    a) Miotics to reduce pupil size
    b) Larger optical zone and larger lens diameter
    c) Smaller optical zone and smaller lens diameter
    d) Larger optical zone and smaller lens diameter

116. **If the pupil dilates into the peripheral curves of a rigid lens, the patient probably will notice:**
    a) Vision is clearer right after a blink, then blurs
    b) Vision is blurred right after a blink, then clears
    c) Blurred vision due to corneal edema
    d) Light streamers (flare)

117. **An eye is considered "dry" if the tear breakup time (BUT) is:**
    a) 10 seconds or less
    b) 15 to 25 seconds
    c) 30 to 40 seconds
    d) Over 45 seconds

118. **A hydrophilic/soft lens will react to a dry eye:**
    a) By drying it further as the lens draws moisture into itself
    b) By restoring the tear balance
    c) By releasing water content from the lens onto the eye
    d) With excessive movement

119. **Fitting a dry eye with a soft lens can be difficult because:**
    a) Tear supplements cannot be used with soft lenses
    b) The lens will move excessively
    c) The diameter of the lens will change as it dries
    d) The optical properties of the lens will change as it dries

120. **The patient with excess tear secretion may experience:**
    a) "Sucked on" lens syndrome
    b) Increased risk of neovascularization
    c) Excess lens movement
    d) Circumcorneal indentation

121. **Which adaptation may need to be made when fitting rigid lenses on a patient with dry eyes?**
    a) Insertion and removal with a plunger only
    b) Enzyme cleaning twice a week instead of once
    c) Less frequent blinking
    d) Longer period to build up to full-time wear

122. **Problems with PMMA interpalpebral lenses include:**
    a) Lid bumping and flare
    b) Apical staining and flattening
    c) Excessive movement and poor centration
    d) Lens-induced astigmatism and reduced visual acuity

123. **Patients with exophthalmos:**
    a) May not be comfortable with a rigid lens
    b) May not be comfortable with a soft lens
    c) Should be fit with an interpalpebral fit rigid lens
    d) Should not wear contacts at all due to dryness

124. **You are using the slit lamp to evaluate a patient with rigid contacts. When the patient blinks, sometimes the upper lid grabs the lens so that the lens rides too high. At other times, the upper lid pushes the lens down. What may cause this to happen?**
    a) The lens diameter is too small
    b) The lens diameter is too large
    c) The lids are too tight
    d) The lids are too lax

125. **Matching (one answer only).**

Fluorescein patterns:	Likely cause:
Horizontal band	a) Overwear
Vertical band	b) Dryness
3 and 9 o'clock staining	c) Foreign body under lens
Diffuse staining	d) Proper fit
Dense apical staining	e) Lens too steep/too much vault
Diffuse apical staining	f) With-the-rule astigmatism
Zigzags	g) Against-the-rule astigmatism
Arc stain	h) Poor insertion/poor blend
Pooling under lens center	i) Lens/cornea contact (keratoconus)
Pooling under lens periphery	j) Edge stand-off/too flat
No stain under lens	k) Chemical/solution sensitivity
No stain in intermediate zone	l) "Sucked on" lens

126. **Which of the following statements about vertex distance is correct?**
    a) Myopes may require more minus power in a soft lens than in spectacles
    b) Hyperopes may require less plus power in a soft lens than in spectacles
    c) Aphakes may require less plus power in a soft lens than in spectacles
    d) Hyperopes may require more plus power in a soft lens than in spectacles

127. **At what power threshold should you begin adjusting the contact lens power for vertex distance?**
    a) 1.00 diopter
    b) 2.00 diopters
    c) 4.00 diopters
    d) 6.00 diopters

128. **In calculating the power for a rigid lens, one must:**
    a) First transpose the prescription into plus cylinder form
    b) First transpose the prescription into minus cylinder form
    c) Calculate the spherical equivalent
    d) Always compensate for vertex distance

129. **The power of a spherical rigid lens (under 4.0 diopters) fit on K:**
    a) Must be adjusted according to the K reading
    b) Is the spherical element of the refractometric measurement
    c) Is the spherical equivalent of the refractometric measurement
    d) Varies according to the lens diameter

130. **The refractometric measurement is - 2.50 - 1.00 X 180. The K readings are 42.00/43.00. You have elected to fit a rigid lens with a base curve of 42.5. What power should you order?**
    a) -3.00
    b) -2.00
    c) -2.50
    d) -3.50

131. **Selecting the power of a soft spherical contact lens is based on:**
    a) The spherical element found on refractometry
    b) The cylindrical element found on refractometry
    c) The spherical equivalent of the refractometric measurement
    d) The refractometric and keratometric measurements

132. **To obtain the spherical equivalent:**
    a) Add half of the sphere to the cylinder algebraically, keeping the cylinder
    b) Add half of the cylinder to the sphere algebraically, keeping the cylinder
    c) Add half of the sphere to the cylinder algebraically, deleting the cylinder
    d) Add half of the cylinder to the sphere algebraically, deleting the cylinder

133. **You want to fit a spherical soft contact. The refractometric measurement is -3.00 + 1.00 X 180. Your lens choice is:**
    a) - 3.00 sphere
    b) - 3.50 sphere
    c) - 2.00 sphere
    d) - 2.50 sphere

134. **You plan to fit a soft toric contact lens. Which of the following is true regarding the refractometric measurement?**
    a) It must be converted to plus cylinder
    b) You will use the spherical equivalent
    c) You want the patient to accept the most cylinder power possible
    d) You want the patient to accept the least cylinder power possible

135. **Over-refractometry of a contact lens is useful in fine tuning:**
    a) Lens power
    b) Lens diameter
    c) Lens centration
    d) Lens base curve

136. **When performing over-refractometry of a contact lens, it is important to:**
    a) Check for residual astigmatism first
    b) Check for a reading add first
    c) Subtract the least amount of sphere that you can
    d) Reduce plus power as much as possible

137. **When taking a refractometric measurement over a contact lens of a patient over 40 years old:**
    a) First find out how the lens is corrected for presbyopia
    b) Measure each eye for distance only
    c) Measure each eye for near only
    d) Measure the right eye for distance and the left eye for near

138. **Residual astigmatism in an otherwise successfully fit contact lens patient is usually generated by:**
    a) The tear film
    b) The cornea
    c) The crystalline lens
    d) The retina

139. **If the refractometric measurement over a spherical soft contact shows uncorrected astigmatism of 0.50 D or less:**
    a) A toric lens should be tried
    b) Refit, using spherical equivalent
    c) A rigid lens should be recommended
    d) In general this can be ignored

140. **A 25-year-old patient was prescribed a -1.75 sphere contact lens for the right eye and a -2.50 sphere contact lens for the left. He comes in complaining that the vision in the left eye is blurry. You measure his visual acuity at 20/20 OD and 20/40 OS. Slit lamp exam is clear. Over-refractometry shows +0.75 sphere OD = 20/20 and -0.75 sphere OS = 20/20. What happened?**
    a) The patient was prescribed the wrong lenses
    b) The patient has developed corneal edema in the right eye
    c) The patient has developed a cataract in the left eye
    d) The patient has switched (crossed) the lenses

141. **Your patient, who wears gas permeable contacts, usually sees 20/20. Today she sees 20/40 OD and 20/30 OS. Over-refractometry does not improve her vision. Up to this point you only have checked vision and done the over-refractometry. What is a logical next step?**
    a) Ask the physician to see her because she must have pathology
    b) Try the lenses in the opposite eye to see if she mixed them up
    c) Examine the patient with the slit lamp (lenses on)
    d) Examine the patient with the slit lamp (lenses off)

142. **The most pressing need for contact lenses in pediatrics is:**
    a) Unilateral aphakia
    b) Bilateral aphakia
    c) Strabismus
    d) Bilateral high myopia

143. **The success of pediatric contact lens wear lies largely with:**
    a) The fitter
    b) The child
    c) The parent
    d) The lens manufacturer

144. **The lens material of choice for infantile aphakia is:**
    a) PMMA
    b) Silicone
    c) HEMA soft
    d) Gas permeable

145. **Considerations when selecting a soft lens for an aphakic pediatric eye include all of the following *except*:**
    a) Steeper base curves
    b) Smaller diameter
    c) Higher powers
    d) Smaller optic zone

146. **An aphakic infant usually is fit with a power:**
    a) Based on near correction
    b) Based on distance correction
    c) Reducing plus to encourage accommodation
    d) On the minus side so he can "grow" into it

147. **Astigmatism in an infant wearing contact lenses may be addressed by all of the following *except*:**
    a) A toric lens
    b) A spherical contact with spectacle overcorrection
    c) Spherical equivalent in a spherical contact
    d) Accepting a less than ideal visual acuity

148. **The main advantage of fitting the small child with soft extended wear lenses is:**
    a) They are more durable
    b) They alleviate daily handling for the parents
    c) They are easier to insert and remove than a rigid lens
    d) They have a lower loss rate

149. **Regarding lens handling in a child patient:**
    a) The child should be taught to handle the lenses around age 10 or 12
    b) The child should be taught to insert and remove the lenses as soon as possible
    c) The parents should continue handling the lenses as long as possible
    d) The fitter should handle the lenses as long as possible

150. **Patients who work around smoke, dust, and chemical fumes should be told:**
    a) They are not good candidates for contact lenses
    b) They should wear rigid lenses, which will not absorb fumes
    c) They should not wear contacts at work
    d) They should change jobs if they want to wear contacts

151. **A rigid lens might be contraindicated in a patient who:**
    a) Plays contact sports
    b) Is presbyopic
    c) Has mild problems with manual dexterity
    d) Is compulsive about his vision

152. **Which patient might you logically want to discourage from wearing contact lenses?**
    a) A 65-year-old aphake who has worn glasses for 12 years
    b) A 35-year-old emmetrope who wants to change her eye color
    c) A 50-year-old emmetrope
    d) A moderately myopic teen

153. **All of the following might contraindicate contact lens wear *except*:**
    a) History of Herpetic keratitis
    b) History of episcleritis
    c) Pinguecula with history of inflammation
    d) Pterygium

154. **Your prospective contact lens patient has glaucoma and uses Propine. She should be told that:**
    a) She is not a good candidate for contact lenses
    b) She'll have to switch to another glaucoma medication if she wears contacts
    c) The drops will have no effect on contact lenses of any type
    d) She should be fit with rigid lenses

155. **In which of the following would contact lenses be contraindicated?**
    a) A patient who has had a cataract removed with an IOL implant
    b) A patient who has had glaucoma filtration surgery
    c) A patient who has had refractive surgery
    d) A patient who has had a corneal graft for keratoconus

156. **All of the following are associated with dry eye and may render a patient a poor contact lens candidate *except*:**
    a) Rheumatoid arthritis
    b) Diabetes
    c) Menopause
    d) Use of allergy medications

157. **A good rule of thumb when instructing patients regarding contact lenses is to:**
    a) Provide a training session offering oral and written instruction
    b) Provide written instruction and instruct the patient to call with questions
    c) Provide a training session and oral instruction
    d) Develop a support group where successful lens wearers teach others

158. **The first rule to teach patients about handling contact lenses is:**
    a) Always use a mirror
    b) Work over a clean surface
    c) Always wash hands first
    d) Never touch the lens itself

159. **Before inserting a soft lens, the patient should make sure it is not inverted. This can be done by:**
    a) Visual inspection or the taco test
    b) Visual inspection or the jelly roll test
    c) Inserting the lens in an inversion tester
    d) Viewing the lens's reverse image in the mirror

160. **To insert a soft lens:**
    a) The lens should be dry and the finger wet
    b) The lens and finger should be dry
    c) The lens should be wet and the finger dry
    d) The lens and finger should be wet

161. **When first learning to insert contact lenses, it is helpful for the patient to use the nondominant hand:**
    a) To immobilize the upper lid
    b) To insert the contact
    c) To pull down the lower lid
    d) The right hand should always be used to insert the lens

162. **The patient should be instructed to place the lens:**
    a) Directly on the cornea
    b) On the inferior sclera, then slide it up
    c) On the margin of the lower lid
    d) On the nasal sclera, then slide it over

163. **Soft lenses are most easily removed by:**
    a) Using a plunger cup
    b) Blinking them out
    c) Squeezing them out
    d) Pinching them out

164. **Damage to soft contact lenses is frequently caused by:**
    a) Pinching them out
    b) Rolling them between the fingers
    c) Long fingernails
    d) Defective materials

165. **Rigid lenses are often removed by blinking them out. For this technique to work:**
    a) The lens should be moved onto the sclera first
    b) The lens must be centered on the eye
    c) The patient must flip the edge of the lens with the finger
    d) The patient must squint and look up

166. **All of the following are helpful/proper techniques for using a plunger to remove a rigid lens** *except*:
    a) Locate the lens on the eye before applying the plunger
    b) Wet the plunger with wetting solution first
    c) Run the plunger over the cornea and sclera to locate a "lost" lens
    d) Carry an extra plunger in pocket or purse for emergency removal

167. **Soft lenses should be cleaned immediately after removal because:**
    a) Grunge is easier to remove at body temperature
    b) The patient might forget to do it later
    c) Grunge is harder to remove once the lens has dried out
    d) Otherwise enzymes are needed

168. **The difference between cleaning and disinfecting is:**
    a) Cleaning is mandatory; disinfecting is optional
    b) Cleaning removes film and debris; disinfecting kills germs
    c) Cleaning kills germs; disinfecting removes film and debris
    d) Cleaning is optional; disinfecting is mandatory

169. **In traditional cleaning systems, when cleaning the lens after removal one should apply cleaner to both surfaces of the lens and:**
    a) Rub it hard between the thumb and index finger
    b) Place the lens in the palm and gently rub with a fingertip
    c) Place the lens in one palm and rub it with the other palm
    d) Rinse the cleaner right off again so it doesn't penetrate the lens

170. **When not being worn, even rigid lenses should be stored in soaking solution because:**
    a) This prevents warpage
    b) This reduces the chances of chipping the lens
    c) This maintains the power of the lens
    d) This maintains the integrity of the plastic

171. **If a gas permeable lens dries out:**
    a) It must be replaced
    b) It can still be worn immediately
    c) It should be soaked for at least 4 hours
    d) It should be soaked for a week before wearing

172. **If the lenses are not going to be worn for a few days:**
    a) Add more soaking solution periodically to keep the lenses covered
    b) Screw the case lid on tight to prevent evaporation
    c) Use only nonpreserved saline as a soak
    d) Change the soaking solution every day to maintain disinfection

173. **Use of lotion or moisturizer before handling lenses, or use of make up, hair spray, or face cream after inserting lenses can cause:**
    a) Lens film
    b) Corneal edema
    c) Degradation of the lens
    d) GPC

174. **The patient asks what he should do if he drops the contact lens into the sink while trying to insert the lens. You tell him:**
    a) Rinse the lens with saline and insert
    b) Rinse the lens with rewetting drops and insert
    c) Clean and disinfect the lens as per solution instructions
    d) Replace the lens

175. **All of the following are true regarding a contact lens case *except*:**
    a) It can be boiled in water
    b) It should be washed weekly with hot water and soap
    c) It should be replaced every couple of months
    d) The interior is disinfected along with the contacts

176. **Wetting solutions are used to:**
    a) Keep lenses sterile while stored in the case
    b) Enable tears to spread evenly on the lens surface
    c) Make the lens resistant to deposit build-up
    d) Prevent scratches on the lens surface

177. **Which of the following is the *least* sterile of these nonapproved, ill-advised, and dangerous re-wetting fluids?**
    a) Saliva
    b) Tap water
    c) Urine
    d) Water from a swimming pool

178. **A surfactant cleaner:**
    a) Is rubbed over the lens surface
    b) Is used to soak the lens
    c) Is used to rewet the lens
    d) Is put in the eye for redness

179. **Enzymatic cleaners are recommended weekly for daily wear soft lenses and gas permeable lenses in order to:**
    a) Sterilize the lenses
    b) Prolong the life of the lens material
    c) Remove protein deposits
    d) Reduce splitting and chipping

180. **Which of the following has been associated with *Acanthamoeba* infections in contact lens wearers?**
    a) Nonpreserved saline
    b) Thimerosal preserved solutions
    c) Homemade saline
    d) Sample bottles of solutions

181. **The "all-in-one" (soaking and wetting) solutions are convenient due to all of the following *except*:**
    a) The cleaning step is eliminated
    b) One can insert the lenses right from the case
    c) One less bottle of solution is required
    d) Lens comfort is increased

182. **Patients should be told that regarding contact lens solution types and brands:**
    a) They can buy whatever is on sale
    b) All brands are mix-and-match
    c) They should only buy from your practice
    d) Some chemicals react negatively with others

183. **Which lens type has a slower schedule for building up wearing time?**
    a) Rigid lens
    b) Daily wear soft lens
    c) Extended wear soft lens
    d) Disposable lens

184. **In general, the recommended upper limit wearing time for daily wear rigid or soft lenses is:**
    a) 8 hours
    b) 10 hours
    c) 15 hours
    d) 20 hours

185. **The suggested first day of wear with rigid lenses is:**
    a) Wear 1 hour, remove 1 hour, wear 1 hour, remove 1 hour, wear 1 hour
    b) Wear 2 hours, remove 3 hours, wear 6 hours
    c) Wear 3 hours, remove 1 hour, wear 3 hours
    d) Wear 5 hours, remove 1 hour, wear 5 hours

186. **After a rigid lens wearer has worked up to 5 to 6 hours a day:**
    a) She is maxed out for the wearing schedule
    b) 1 hour is added every other day
    c) She immediately can increase to 15 hours a day
    d) 2 hours are added every day

187. **Using a proper wearing schedule, a rigid contact lens wearer will work up to full-time wear in about:**
    a) 1 to 2 weeks
    b) 4 to 5 weeks
    c) 8 to 10 weeks
    d) 12 to 15 weeks

188. **The schedule for the first day of wearing soft lenses is:**
    a) Wear 2 hours, remove 1 hour, wear 2 hours
    b) Wear 8 to 10 hours
    c) Wear 15 hours
    d) Wear 1 hour, remove 1 hour, wear 1 hour

189. **Using a proper wearing schedule, a soft lens wearer can build up to full-time wear in approximately:**
    a) 1 week
    b) 3 to 4 weeks
    c) 6 to 8 weeks
    d) 10 to 12 weeks

190. **Symptoms of rigid contact lens overwear (overwear syndrome, or OWS) include all of the following *except*:**
    a) Moderate to severe pain and photophobia
    b) Lid swelling
    c) Discomfort starts immediately after removing lenses
    d) Tearing

191. **The most obvious slit lamp finding in OWS is:**
    a) Apical fluorescein staining
    b) Corneal edema
    c) Corneal neovascularization
    d) Corneal ulceration

192. **The contact lens patient should be told that if the eye ever becomes red or painful, he is to:**
    a) Try another lens
    b) Irrigate the eye
    c) Bear with it
    d) Remove the lens

193. **Corneal edema, sensations of soreness, injection, foggy vision, and ghost images usually indicate:**
    a) A tight-fitting lens
    b) Decentration and corneal exposure
    c) Allergy to soft lens solutions
    d) That the lens is too small and too flat

194. **Under the slit lamp a tight soft contact lens might exhibit all of the following *except*:**
    a) Conjunctival drag
    b) Circumcorneal injection
    c) Edge standoff
    d) Scleral indentation

195. **A patient with a tight soft lens will notice that her vision:**
    a) Is stable
    b) Is clearer in the evening than in the morning
    c) Is clearer just after a blink, then blurs
    d) Is blurred just after a blink, then clears

196. **A tight soft lens can be loosened by:**
    a) Decreasing the diameter or flattening the base curve
    b) Increasing the diameter or steepening the base curve
    c) Increasing the lens vault
    d) Compensating for vertex distance

197. **Your patient complains that he can constantly feel his soft lens in his eye. He also experiences some blurred vision, especially when he moves his eyes around a lot. These are symptoms of:**
    a) A tight lens
    b) A loose lens
    c) Inadequate power
    d) Poor hygiene

198. **Slit lamp examination in the case of a loose soft lens may reveal:**
    a) No movement, decentration, and conjunctival drag
    b) Multiple deposits and "jelly bumps"
    c) Limbal injection, corneal edema, and vascularization
    d) Excessive movement, decentration, edge puckering, and edge standoff

199. **A loose soft lens may be tightened by:**
    a) Decreasing the base curve or decreasing the diameter
    b) Steepening the base curve or increasing the diameter
    c) Removing deposits and instructing the patient on proper lens care
    d) Increasing the power to compensate for vertex distance

200. **Vascularization can result from chronic:**
    a) Hypoxia
    b) Solution sensitivity
    c) Conjunctival injection
    d) GPC

201. **The area of the cornea that most commonly becomes vascularized is the:**
    a) Inferior limbal area
    b) Superior limbal area
    c) 9:00 limbal area
    d) 3:00 limbal area

202. **Which patient is most likely to develop vascularization?**
    a) Moderate myope with extended wear lenses
    b) High myope with gas permeable lenses
    c) Pseudophake with gas permeable lenses
    d) Aphake with extended wear lenses

203. **In a soft lens patient with vascularization, the problem might be remedied by all of the following *except*:**
    a) A looser lens
    b) A change in solutions
    c) A thinner lens
    d) A higher water content

204. **A rigid lens may stimulate vascularization if it:**
    a) Is not cleaned weekly with enzymatic cleaner
    b) Lifts, then slides down a little after each blink
    c) Habitually rides on the central cornea
    d) Habitually rides on the limbus

205. *Pseudomonas* **ulcers are seen more frequently in patients wearing:**
   a) Gas permeable lenses
   b) Extended wear soft lenses
   c) Daily wear soft lenses
   d) Daily wear soft toric lenses

206. A corneal ulcer associated with contact lens wear can be caused by all of the following *except*:
   a) Chemical sensitivity
   b) Infection
   c) Trauma
   d) Hypoxia

207. Corneal ulcers are usually unrelated to use of:
   a) Daily wear soft lenses
   b) Extended wear soft lenses
   c) Extended wear soft lenses removed on a daily basis
   d) Gas permeable rigid lenses

208. Some patients experience reduced vision with their glasses after removing their contact lenses. This can last from several minutes to several weeks, and is known as:
   a) Contact lens blur
   b) Spectacle blur
   c) Overwear syndrome
   d) Corneal edema

209. Spectacle blur is due to:
   a) Corneal edema
   b) Corneal molding
   c) Contact lens overwear
   d) Both a and b

210. The type of lenses most often associated with spectacle blur is:
   a) PMMA rigid lenses
   b) Gas permeable lenses
   c) Daily wear soft contact lenses
   d) Extended wear soft contact lenses

211. The best solution for spectacle blur is to fit the patient with:
   a) PMMA rigid lenses
   b) Gas permeable lenses
   c) Daily wear soft contact lenses
   d) Extended wear soft contact lenses

212. GPC is suspected to be:
   a) An allergic response
   b) An infection
   c) A response to mechanical irritation
   d) A sign of overwear

213. In addition to mucus formation, itching, and lens intolerance, the hallmark of GPC is:
   a) Corneal ulcers
   b) Inflamed pingueculae
   c) Papillae on the palpebral conjunctiva of the upper lid
   d) Papillae on the bulbar conjunctiva under the upper lid

214. The occurrence of GPC may be increased by wearing a soft lens:
   a) With a diameter less than 12.0 mm
   b) With a diameter over 14.0 mm
   c) That is too flat
   d) That is too loose

215. GPC is the body's response to:
   a) Hypoxia
   b) A warped lens
   c) A torn lens
   d) Protein deposits

216. GPC usually can be managed by:
   a) Switching the patient to a heat disinfection system
   b) Refitting the patient with extended wear lenses
   c) Dispensing new lenses, and using surfactant and enzymatic cleaners regularly
   d) Continuing lens wear while using vasoconstrictor drops

217. The most common symptom of contact lens deposits is:
   a) Foreign body sensation
   b) Corneal edema
   c) Vascularization
   d) Itching and watering

218. "Jelly bumps" on a soft contact lens are actually:
   a) Areas where the lens has dehydrated
   b) Dried mucus
   c) Calcium and lipid deposits
   d) Dried eye ointment

219. A silicone gas permeable lens is prone to:
   a) Waxy deposits
   b) Calcium buildup
   c) Jelly bumps
   d) Dehydration

220. There is some evidence that as deposits form on a lens:
   a) There is a decrease in its water content
   b) There is a decrease in its oxygen transmission
   c) There is an increase in lens dehydration
   d) There is a decrease in lens dehydration

221. Which of the following is *not* true regarding protein build-up on a soft contact lens?
   a) It is a common problem with soft lenses
   b) The deposits can be picked off the lens
   c) Enzyme cleaners can help reduce the problem
   d) Frequent lens changes may be required

222. The most serious aspect of protein build-up on a soft lens (especially an extended wear soft lens) is:
   a) Corneal abrasion
   b) Bacterial growth
   c) It can trigger GPC
   d) Discomfort

223. **Label the following items as: a) May cause discomfort, or b) Unlikely to cause discomfort:**
    A. Vascularization
    B. Adaptation to new lenses
    C. Lens switch
    D. Foreign body
    E. Inverted lens
    F. Vertex distance not accounted for
    G. Corneal abrasion
    H. Incorrect power
    I. GPC
    J. Lens overwear
    K. Corneal edema
    L. Infection
    M. Lens deposits
    N. Tight lens
    O. Loose lens
    P. Change in prescription
    Q. Toxic reaction to solutions
    R. Corneal ulcer
    S. Torn lens
    T. Rigid lens crazing
    U. Smooth lens edges
    V. Fenestrated lens
    W. Limbal touch
    X. Excessive movement

224. **If the fit of a rigid lens looks good after 2 months but the lens is uncomfortable, a logical course of action would be to:**
    a) Switch the patient to soft lenses
    b) Encourage the patient to continue to adapt to the lenses
    c) Suggest enzymatic cleaning twice weekly
    d) Blend curves, roll edges, and polish well

225. **A former PMMA patient who is refit with gas permeable lenses will experience a gradual increase in discomfort before adapting to the lenses. This is due to:**
    a) Increase in corneal hypoxia
    b) Necrosis of the corneal nerve endings
    c) Recovery of the corneal nerve endings
    d) Decrease in corneal sensation

226. **Which of the following would be *most* useful in fitting a keratoconus patient?**
    a) Corneal pachymetry
    b) Corneal topography
    c) Keratometry
    d) Placido's disk

227. **Early keratoconus often may be successfully corrected by:**
    a) Soft lenses and glasses
    b) Thin cut PMMA lenses
    c) McGuire or "nipple" cone contact lenses
    d) "Globus" cone contact lenses

228. Moderate keratoconus of 45.00 to 50.00 may often be fit with:
a) Soft toric lenses
b) Gas permeable lenses
c) McGuire or "nipple" cone contact lenses
d) Soper contact lenses

229. As the cone progresses, rigid lenses are required in order to:
a) Compensate for vertex distance
b) Provide a smooth refractive surface
c) Increase patient comfort
d) Enable the patient to stop wearing glasses

230. An acceptable rigid lens fit on a keratoconus patient includes:
a) A large diameter so the lens almost touches the limbus
b) A steep enough base curve to vault the apex
c) A larger lens diameter and as little movement as possible
d) A smaller lens diameter and minimal apical touch

231. A Soper, McGuire, or "globus" specialty lens might be used in keratoconus cases where:
a) A smaller, flatter lens is needed
b) A larger, steeper lens is needed
c) A steeper lens with good movement is needed
d) A steeper lens with almost no movement is needed

232. Corneal edema is caused by:
a) Excess oxygen permeability
b) Insufficient oxygen
c) Excess carbon dioxide
d) Excess tear production

233. Symptoms of corneal edema include:
a) Blurred vision
b) Rainbows around lights
c) Injection and burning
d) All of the above

234. A patient wearing extended wear contact lenses who develops corneal edema might be managed by:
a) Increasing the lens diameter
b) Trying different water contents
c) Fitting on K
d) Increasing wearing time

235. A patient who is wearing rigid lenses and develops corneal edema might be managed by:
a) Increasing the diameter of the optic zone
b) Steepening the peripheral curve
c) Increasing diameter
d) Improving tear exchange

236. Which of the following statements about salt tablets is correct?
a) Saline for use with soft contact lenses can be made from any USP salt tablets
b) Solution in the saline mixing bottle can be used to rehydrate soft lenses in the eye
c) *Acanthamoeba* keratitis occurs more frequently in patients who make their own saline
d) Saline made from salt tablets is more likely to cause GPC

237. **Patients should be warned *not* to mix and match contact lens solutions because:**
    a) It is easier to contaminate the lenses this way
    b) Expiration dates may not match
    c) This encourages growth of *Pseudomonas*
    d) Certain chemicals and preservatives are not compatible

238. **A common cause of red eyes in contact lens wearers that is sometimes misdiagnosed as tight lens syndrome, conjunctivitis, episcleritis, or other ailments is:**
    a) Chlorhexidine allergy
    b) Using enzyme cleaner without disinfecting
    c) Thimerosal allergy
    d) *Acanthamoeba* contamination

239. **The contact lens patient with suspected chemical sensitivity should be told to:**
    a) Discontinue lens wear
    b) Clean and store lenses in unpreserved saline
    c) Use unpreserved solutions and try a hydrogen peroxide disinfection system
    d) Try solutions until he finds one that does not cause the reaction

240. **Aphakic rigid lenses will often center better if:**
    a) A hyperflange is incorporated into the lens design
    b) The lens is ordered in a single cut design
    c) The lens is fit on K
    d) A myoflange is incorporated into the lens design

241. **All of the following modifications can be performed on a rigid lens *except*:**
    a) Increase diameter
    b) Rebevel
    c) Blend
    d) Buff or taper edge

242. **Which of the following situations can be remedied by modifying a rigid lens?**
    a) 42-year-old just noticing presbyopia
    b) Hyperope fit with a +2.50 sph, now needs a +3.00 sph
    c) Hyperope fit with a +2.50 sph, now needs a +2.00 sph
    d) Myope fit with a -2.50 sph, now needs a -2.00 sph

243. **If a patient is refit with a flatter lens:**
    a) Adjust the power by adding minus
    b) Adjust the power by adding plus
    c) Adjust the power only if vertex distance is an issue
    d) There is no need to adjust the power at all

244. **Fenestration of a PMMA lens is done in order to:**
    a) Increase oxygen supply to the cornea
    b) Improve tear exchange under the lens
    c) Improve lens movement
    d) Increase patient comfort

245. **Blurred vision due to hypoxia usually:**
    a) Fluctuates throughout the day
    b) Starts as soon as the lenses are inserted but clears later
    c) Starts several hours after the lenses are inserted
    d) Is continuous from the time of insertion to removal

246. **Blurred vision associated with a tight or loose lens:**
    a) Fluctuates throughout the day
    b) Fluctuates with blinking
    c) Starts several hours after the lenses are inserted
    d) Is always accompanied by redness and discomfort

247. **Vision that is clear initially after a blink but then blurs may be associated with:**
    a) Incorrect power
    b) Excessive lens movement
    c) Sucked-on lens syndrome
    d) Too large an optical zone

248. **Blurred vision that occurs after prolonged reading may be due to:**
    a) Presbyopia
    b) Lack of tearing
    c) Excessive blinking
    d) An out-of-date prescription

249. **In soft lens wearers, the most common cause of blurred vision is:**
    a) An inverted lens
    b) A chemical allergy
    c) Excessive movement
    d) Lens dehydration

250. **Your contact lens patient complains of cloudy vision. What is the most important thing to determine?**
    a) Tear break-up time
    b) If the problem is corneal or contact-lens related
    c) How old the lenses are
    d) Whether the patient is cleaning the lenses properly

251. **When reading the power of a high plus rigid contact lens, it is important to know:**
    a) If it is front or back vertex power
    b) If it is truncated
    c) What material it is made of
    d) Its radius of curvature

252. **To read the back vertex power (BVD) of a rigid lens on the lensometer:**
    a) Place the convex surface toward the lens stop
    b) Place the concave surface toward the lens stop
    c) Read convex and concave surfaces and subtract them
    d) Read convex and concave surfaces and add them

253. **When reading the power of a toric lens, one must make sure to:**
    a) Align the truncation or markings so that they match the axis that was ordered
    b) Align the truncation or markings 90 degrees away from the axis that was ordered
    c) Align the truncation or markings at the top of the lens
    d) Align the truncation or markings at the bottom of the lens

254. **The Tori-check® device can be used to verify:**
    a) Toric alignment
    b) Toric lens balance
    c) Toric lens power and axis
    d) Toric lens axis

255. **The power of a soft contact lens can be measured:**
     a) Soft lenses are not verified because they are labeled by the manufacturer
     b) Soft lenses are not verified because they dry out too quickly
     c) By blotting and placing it on the lensometer
     d) Only by placing it in a wet cell and reading on the lensometer

256. **The radiuscope is used to:**
     a) Measure the curvature of the peripheral cornea
     b) Measure the base curve of a rigid lens
     c) Check the calibration of the keratometer
     d) Help fit toric lenses with greater precision

257. **To read the base curve with a radiuscope, the contact is floated on a drop of water:**
     a) On its edge
     b) Convex side up
     c) Concave side up
     d) Concave side down

258. **Number the following steps of using the radiuscope in chronological order:**
     ___Focus the spoke image and set the measuring scale to zero
     ___Raise the microscope until the aerial image is seen
     ___Raise the microscope and focus the measuring scale
     ___Take the reading
     ___Lower the microscope until the lamp filament image is seen
     ___Center the contact and lens mount
     ___Lower the microscope further until the spoke target is seen

259. **If, after finding and focusing the spoke image, the radiuscope's measuring scale cannot be set to zero, you should set it to the next whole number: +1.00. At this setting, what will you need to do to the final reading?**
     a) Subtract 1.00 mm
     b) Add 1.00 mm
     c) Read it directly off the scale
     d) One can always set the measuring scale to zero

260. **You have finished reading the base curve and see the image in Figure 5-1. The patient has flat, spherical K readings, and the refractometric measurement is -2.50 + 0.50 X 180. The appearance of the target is due to the fact that:**
    a) The lens is toric
    b) The lens is drying out
    c) The lens is too steep
    d) The lens is warped

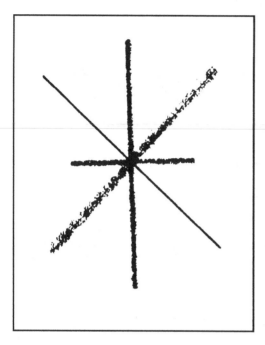

Figure 5-1. Reprinted with permission from Rakow PL. *Contact Lenses*. Thorofare, NJ: SLACK Incorporated; 1988.

261. **To evaluate a lens for warpage, one should view the radiuscope mires:**
    a) Of the filament image
    b) Of the lens profile image
    c) Of the real image
    d) Of the aerial image

262. **The base curve of a soft lens:**
    a) Need not be measured because it comes labeled by the manufacturer
    b) Cannot be measured because the lens dries out too quickly
    c) Can be measured by placing the lens on a plastic template
    d) Can be measured only by using a Soft Lens Analyzer®

263. **When measuring the diameter of a rigid lens using a V-groove diameter gauge, one should:**
    a) Gently place the lens on top of the ruler
    b) Push the lens as far into the groove as it will go
    c) Let the lens roll into place
    d) Hydrate the lens well

264. The lens diameter is taken from the V-groove diameter gauge by:
a) Taking the reading directly off the dial
b) Reading the scale mark on the left side of the lens
c) Reading the scale mark on the right side of the lens
d) Reading the scale mark nearest the center of the lens

265. The lens diameter of a soft lens can be measured:
a) With a V-groove diameter gauge
b) By setting the lens gently on a magnifier with a millimeter scale
c) By pressing the lens down flat on a magnifier with a millimeter scale
d) Only with a Soft Lens Analyzer

266. A thickness gauge is used to measure the central thickness of:
a) Disposable lenses
b) Extended wear soft lenses
c) Rigid lenses
d) Bandage lenses

267. Before using the thickness gauge, one must:
a) Hydrate the contact lens
b) Calibrate the gauge for the lens material
c) Set the eyepiece to one's refractive error
d) Set the gauge to the zero setting

268. The edges of a soft contact lens can be evaluated:
a) By viewing with a magnifier
b) Only by using a Soft Lens Analyzer
c) By using a profile analyzer
d) With a lensometer

269. The edges of a rigid contact lens can be evaluated by using a/an:
a) Radiuscope
b) Profile analyzer
c) Lensometer
d) Edging gauge

270. The profile image of a rigid contact having smooth and blended zones will:
a) Look serrated
b) Show definite demarcations between curves
c) Have a "ski" contour
d) Look like a lightning bolt

Chapter 6

Intermediate
Tonometry

1. **The aqueous humor is produced by the:**
   a) Ciliary muscle
   b) Ciliary body
   c) Trabecular meshwork
   d) Iris

2. **The composition of the aqueous is most like:**
   a) Blood plasma
   b) Tears
   c) Saliva
   d) Mucus

3. **The flow of aqueous in the eye follows this pattern:**
   a) Angle, posterior chamber, pupil, anterior chamber
   b) Angle, anterior chamber, pupil, posterior chamber
   c) Pupil, posterior chamber, anterior chamber, angle
   d) Posterior chamber, pupil, anterior chamber, angle

4. **As it exits the eye, aqueous humor flows in this pattern:**
   a) Canal of Schlemm, trabecular meshwork, episcleral arteries
   b) Trabecular meshwork, canal of Schlemm, episcleral veins
   c) Trabecular meshwork, nasolacrimal duct, episcleral arteries
   d) Canal of Schlemm, episcleral veins, trabecular meshwork

5. **Intraocular pressure (IOP) is determined by:**
   a) Systolic and diastolic blood pressure
   b) Rate of aqueous production and resistance to outflow
   c) Pressure in the ophthalmic artery and vein
   d) Cranial pressure transferred to the eye through the optic nerve

6. **Reduction and control of elevated IOP is based on:**
   a) Lowering the diastolic and systolic blood pressure
   b) Lowering cranial pressure
   c) Increasing aqueous production and/or decreasing outflow
   d) Decreasing aqueous production and/or increasing outflow

7. **Which of the following regarding aqueous and IOP is *not* true?**
   a) IOP is generally higher in the morning than in the evening
   b) IOP is slightly higher in the posterior chamber than in the anterior chamber
   c) Aqueous has no effect on the optical system of the eye
   d) Aqueous provides nutrition and waste removal for internal ocular structures

8. **Risk factors for glaucoma include all of the following *except*:**
   a) Hypertension
   b) Positive family history
   c) African-American heritage
   d) Ocular trauma

9. **Glaucoma screening programs are plagued by all of the following *except*:**
   a) Air-puff tonometry, commonly used for screening, is not the most accurate method
   b) A single, normal pressure reading does not necessarily indicate the absence of glaucoma
   c) It generates public interest in the disorder and its treatment
   d) Some normal pressures register as high and some high pressures read normal

10. **The most common type of glaucoma is:**
    a) Congenital
    b) Secondary
    c) Open-angle
    d) Angle-closure

11. **Glaucoma is classically characterized by the triad of increased IOP, visual field damage, and:**
    a) Pigment in the trabecular meshwork
    b) Decreased facility outflow
    c) Fluctuating visual acuity
    d) Optic nerve head damage

12. **In addition to tonometry, the diagnosis of glaucoma may be based on all of the following tests** *except***:**
    a) Ophthalmoscopy
    b) Gonioscopy
    c) Retinoscopy
    d) Perimetry

13. **Gonioscopy is used to evaluate:**
    a) The angle structures
    b) The optic nerve
    c) Peripheral vision
    d) Corneal edema

14. **Vision lost by glaucoma damage:**
    a) Can be recovered if the IOP is brought under control
    b) Can be recovered if laser treatment is used
    c) Can be recovered with certain topical or oral medications
    d) Generally cannot be recovered

15. **The diurnal curve of IOP in a glaucoma patient:**
    a) May vary by 4 mm
    b) May vary up to 10 mm
    c) Is less than in an eye without glaucoma
    d) Produces IOP that is lower in the morning

16. **Symptoms and signs for acute angle-closure glaucoma may include all of the following** *except***:**
    a) Severe pain
    b) Decreased vision
    c) Vomiting/nausea
    d) Miotic pupil

17. **A patient phones in with a painful red eye. In addition to an angle-closure glaucoma attack, you must ask questions to discern whether the patient might, instead, have any of the following** *except***:**
    a) Iritis
    b) Conjunctivitis
    c) Subconjunctival hemorrhage
    d) Keratoconjunctivitis

18. **In angle-closure glaucoma:**
    a) The iris closes off the anterior chamber angle
    b) There is a sudden surge of aqueous production
    c) A miotic pupil prevents aqueous passage
    d) Corneal edema closes off the anterior chamber angle

19. **Emergency treatment during an angle-closure glaucoma attack includes pressure lowering medications and:**
    a) Miotics
    b) Mydriatics
    c) Antibiotics
    d) Corticosteroids

20. **All of the following may trigger an angle-closure glaucoma attack *except*:**
    a) Being dilated in the office
    b) Being in a dark room
    c) Sudden exposure to bright light
    d) Sitting in a movie theater

21. **Which of the following conditions gives a higher risk for developing an angle-closure glaucoma attack?**
    a) High hyperopia
    b) High myopia
    c) Aphakia
    d) Keratoconus

22. **The appearance of halos around lights during an attack of angle-closure glaucoma is due to:**
    a) Lens edema
    b) Corneal edema
    c) Vitreous hemorrhage
    d) Optic nerve damage

23. **All of the following are true regarding open-angle glaucoma *except*:**
    a) It is more prevalent in the African-American population
    b) It can be cured
    c) Optic nerve damage cannot be reversed
    d) It might be controlled with a single medication

24. **The dangerous element of open-angle glaucoma is:**
    a) Pain
    b) Rapid, irreversible visual loss
    c) Lack of symptoms
    d) Lack of signs

25. **In open-angle glaucoma:**
    a) The iris blocks off the angle structures
    b) The pressure damages the ciliary body
    c) The open-angle allows too much aqueous to drain out
    d) The angle looks normal

26. A patient known to have open-angle glaucoma:
   a) Should not be dilated
   b) Should have his pressures checked with an air-puff tonometer
   c) Should be checked annually with confrontation fields
   d) Needs annual dilation, gonioscopy, and formal visual fields

27. A patient in the end stages of open-angle glaucoma:
   a) May have a small island of vision temporally
   b) May have a small island of vision centrally
   c) May have a small island of vision nasally
   d) Still has enough peripheral vision to get around

28. A patient with open-angle glaucoma has missed an appointment for a pressure check. The practice should:
   a) Wait for the patient to call and reschedule, then emphasize the importance of IOP checks
   b) Inform the patient's relatives, and stress the importance of having IOP checks
   c) Have the pharmacist ask the patient to call the office when medication needs to be refilled
   d) Contact the patient immediately to reschedule, emphasizing the importance of IOP checks

29. The physiologic cup of the optic nerve:
   a) Is an abnormal finding in glaucoma
   b) Represents the normal opening in the sclera
   c) Is the area of finest central vision
   d) Is a normal depression in the macular area

30. In glaucoma, the term "cupping" refers to:
   a) A pale optic disc
   b) A decrease and "pinching" in the size of the physiologic cup
   c) An enlargement and "caving in" of the physiologic cup
   d) Dips in the retinal veins and arteries

31. A comparison of the proportion of damaged disc to visually functioning disc is termed:
   a) Abnormal retinal correspondence
   b) The cup-to-disc ratio
   c) The AC/A ratio
   d) The glaucoma ratio

32. A large cup would be represented by:
   a) 0.2
   b) 0.9
   c) 20/400
   d) 30 mm Hg

33. The first area of the optic nerve to be damaged by elevated IOP is often:
   a) The center of the disc
   b) The interior of the disc
   c) The nasal side of the disc
   d) The upper and lower portions of the rim

34. The areas of optic nerve damage directly relate to:
   a) The visual field pattern
   b) The diurnal curve of IOP
   c) Laser treatment
   d) Areas of neovascularization

35. **Patients should be told that their glaucoma medications:**
    a) Need not be used on the day of their appointment
    b) Will cure the condition
    c) Do not need to be refilled
    d) Should be continued until told otherwise

36. **Reasons that a patient fails to take his medications properly include all of the following *except*:**
    a) Lack of symptoms suggesting he has a disease
    b) Side effects of glaucoma medications
    c) He understands the serious nature of the disease
    d) Lack of visual improvement from the medication

37. **The first choice of medicinal treatment for open-angle glaucoma is usually:**
    a) Oral
    b) Topical
    c) Subconjunctival injection
    d) Intravenous

38. **All of the following are employed in reducing IOP *except*:**
    a) Carbonic anhydrase inhibitors (CAIs)
    b) Steroids
    c) Beta blockers
    d) Prostaglandin analogues

39. **Which condition probably would cause the most visual problems from miotics taken for glaucoma?**
    a) Posterior subcapsular cataract
    b) Peripheral cortical cataract
    c) Aphakia
    d) Being over age 65

40. **The topical medication of first choice in treating open-angle glaucoma is often:**
    a) Epinephrine derivatives
    b) Osmotics
    c) Beta blockers
    d) Miotics

41. **In general, which of the following would likely *not* be given to a patient with asthma or other respiratory problems?**
    a) Osmotics
    b) Beta blockers
    c) Prostaglandin analogues
    d) Miotics

42. **When glycerin is given orally to lower IOP in cases of angle-closure glaucoma:**
    a) The patient is told to drink it quickly
    b) It is served over ice mixed with juice
    c) It is given as a time-release capsule
    d) The patient is told to hold the tablet under the tongue

43. **Laser surgery for open-angle glaucoma mainly involves:**
    a) Treating the trabecular meshwork
    b) Treating the ciliary body
    c) Treating the canal of Schlemm
    d) Sealing the puncta

44. **In angle-closure glaucoma, a laser is used to create a(n):**
    a) Iridotomy
    b) Peripheral iridectomy
    c) Sector iridectomy
    d) Iris ablation

45. **The primary goal in most every procedure for angle-closure glaucoma is to:**
    a) Enlarge the pupil
    b) Prevent angle-closure
    c) Provide for aqueous flow between the chambers
    d) Reduce aqueous production

46. **A potential complication or side effect of laser treatment is:**
    a) Elevated blood pressure
    b) Corneal neovascularization
    c) Elevated IOP
    d) Retinal neovascularization

47. **The surgical procedure that creates an external drainage area via a pathway to the anterior chamber is a(n):**
    a) Trabeculectomy
    b) Cycloablation
    c) Iridotomy
    d) Iridectomy

48. **In some aqueous draining procedures, aqueous is drained from the anterior chamber to an area under the conjunctiva. This area is known as a/an:**
    a) Subconjunctival canal
    b) Bleb
    c) Pinguecula
    d) Iris cyst

49. **In the procedure described above, the most common reason for failure is:**
    a) Swelling
    b) Elevated IOP
    c) Scarring
    d) Cystic fibrosis

50. **In an effort to reduce the amount of aqueous produced, surgical procedures may be used to:**
    a) Destroy the ciliary body
    b) Stimulate the ciliary body
    c) Open the trabecular meshwork
    d) Destroy the trabecular meshwork

51. **Indentation tonometry measures IOP by measuring the force:**
    a) It takes to equalize the eye's internal pressure
    b) Exerted on the instrument by the eye
    c) It takes to flatten an area of the cornea
    d) It takes to indent the cornea

52. **When the Schiotz tonometer is applied to the eye:**
    a) The aqueous remains constant
    b) The aqueous is displaced
    c) More aqueous is produced
    d) The scleral buckles

53. **Which of the following statements is *not* true?**
    a) The Schiotz tonometer may be sterilized by flame or autoclave
    b) IOP can be read directly off of the Schiotz tonometer's scale
    c) The correct calibration reading for a Schiotz tonometer is zero.
    d) The Schiotz tonometer weights are not interchangeable between instruments

54. **Which of the following may result in false low readings in Schiotz tonometry?**
    a) Young or highly myopic eyes
    b) Young or highly hyperopic eyes
    c) Presbyopic or geriatric eyes
    d) Albino or light colored eyes

55. **A false reading with the Schiotz tonometer can also result:**
    a) If the patient squeezes his eyelids
    b) If the instrument abrades the cornea
    c) If there is a rush of fluid into the anterior chamber
    d) If the weight disc used is too heavy

56. **Repeating measurements on the same eye with a Schiotz tonometer can result in:**
    a) Artificially increased IOP
    b) Artificially decreased IOP
    c) Decreased scleral rigidity
    d) A diurnal curve in IOP

57. **Which of the following does *not* cause a false reading with indentation tonometry?**
    a) Not compensating for an eye with high astigmatism
    b) Repeated measurements on the same patient
    c) Patient squeezing her eyelids during the measurement
    d) Young or highly myopic eyes

58. **Scleral rigidity refers to:**
    a) The amount of distensibility, or "give", of the sclera
    b) The resistance of the sclera to the pressure of the aqueous humor
    c) The amount of pressure required to indent or flatten the sclera
    d) The resistance of the sclera to the pressure of the vitreous humor

59. **An eye with high elasticity:**
    a) Has no scleral rigidity
    b) Has a high scleral rigidity
    c) Has a low scleral rigidity
    d) Has elevated IOP

60. Scleral rigidity is a factor in indentation tonometry because:
   a) The pressure of the instrument displaces aqueous
   b) The pressure of the instrument distends the extraocular muscles
   c) Holding the patient's eyelids open puts pressure on the sclera
   d) The pressure of the instrument distends the cornea

61. In the normal eye, during indentation tonometry:
   a) The ocular structures and sclera "give" as a response to the displacement of aqueous
   b) The ocular structures and sclera resist the displacement of aqueous
   c) Repeated measurements can lead to "toughening" of the ocular structures and sclera
   d) The ocular structures and sclera are unaffected by the displacement of aqueous

62. In indentation tonometry, an erroneous reading due to scleral rigidity may be identified by:
   a) Taking readings at different times of day
   b) Having the patient sit up for the reading
   c) Taking two readings with different weights
   d) Eliminating the use of topical anesthetic

63. When measuring the same eye with the Schiotz tonometer using different weights, an error due to scleral rigidity is suspected if:
   a) There is a difference of 3 mm between the readings
   b) There is a difference of 1 mm between the readings
   c) The reading taken with the patient sitting up is lower
   d) The morning reading is higher than the afternoon reading

64. If scleral rigidity may be causing inaccurate IOP measurements, one should:
   a) Recheck the patient's IOP in the morning
   b) Recheck the patient's IOP with an applanation tonometer
   c) Gently press on the globe to equalize scleral distention
   d) Tell the patient to hold still during the measurement

65. The applanation tonometer is preferred in cases of low scleral rigidity because:
   a) It does not displace an appreciable amount of aqueous
   b) It does not indent the cornea
   c) It is performed with the patient in a seated position
   d) Topical anesthetic is used

66. The Schiotz tonometer should be cleaned:
   a) At the beginning of each day
   b) At the end of each day
   c) Between each patient
   d) When it appears dirty

67. The barrel of the Schiotz is cleaned:
   a) With a pipe cleaner dipped in alcohol or ether
   b) With a pipe cleaner dipped in boiled water
   c) With a pipe cleaner dipped in iodine
   d) By pouring alcohol through it

68. Wiping the parts of a Schiotz tonometer with alcohol or ether:
   a) Effectively sterilizes it
   b) Effectively cleans it
   c) Can cause the numbers to fade
   d) Can eventually cause rust

69. **The cleaned plunger of the Schiotz tonometer should be reinserted:**
    a) With the fingers
    b) Using a tissue or gloves
    c) Only right before use
    d) The plunger is not removed

70. **The Schiotz tonometer should be allowed to thoroughly dry after proper cleaning before the next use because:**
    a) This kills bacteria
    b) This kills the AIDS virus
    c) A drippy tonometer is uncomfortable to the patient
    d) Cleaning chemicals are toxic to the cornea

71. **All of the following may be used to sterilize the Schiotz tonometer *except*:**
    a) An alcohol wipe
    b) Ultraviolet sterilizer
    c) Soaking in a 1:10 bleach solution
    d) Use of a flame or burner

72. **Which of the following is a disadvantage of the Schiotz tonometer?**
    a) It is expensive
    b) It is difficult to use
    c) It is difficult to calibrate
    d) Scleral rigidity can cause inaccuracy

73. **The advantages of the Schiotz tonometer include:**
    a) It is highly accurate
    b) It requires no anesthetic
    c) It can be used at bedside
    d) It does not need to be cleaned

74. **Before use, the Schiotz tonometer must be calibrated. This is done by:**
    a) Taking a preliminary reading on the patient
    b) Holding the instrument against your finger
    c) Holding the instrument against a flat surface
    d) Holding the instrument on a factory metal test block

75. **If the Schiotz does not zero out when calibrated, the assistant may:**
    a) Bend the needle so it reads zero
    b) Deduct the difference from the patient's reading
    c) Add the difference to the patient's reading
    d) Return it to the manufacturer

76. **Patient position for Schiotz tonometry is:**
    a) Sitting up to the slit lamp
    b) Sitting up in the exam chair
    c) Lying back in the exam chair
    d) Sitting at a 45 degree angle

77. **When holding the lids open for indentation tonometry, it is important to:**
    a) Apply even pressure on the entire eye
    b) Press the lids back onto the globe
    c) Put pressure only on the bony orbit
    d) Use a lid speculum

78. **The Schiotz tonometer is applied to the eye:**
    a) At a 45 degree angle
    b) Parallel to the floor
    c) Perpendicular to the central cornea
    d) Perpendicular to the sclera

79. **In properly aligned Schiotz tonometry:**
    a) There are no factors that affect the IOP
    b) The needle may pulsate slightly with the heartbeat
    c) The needle may pulsate slightly when the patient breathes
    d) Accuracy is assured

80. **When the Schiotz needle pulsates, the IOP:**
    a) Is the lowest of the readings
    b) Is the highest of the readings
    c) Is the difference between the two readings
    d) Is at midpoint between the two readings

81. **In Schiotz tonometry, a high reading on the instrument itself indicates:**
    a) The presence of glaucoma
    b) A high IOP
    c) A low IOP
    d) The weights are inaccurate

82. **If a Schiotz tonometer reading of 2.5 is obtained with the 5.5 weight:**
    a) Use the chart to convert the reading to mm mercury
    b) Remove the weight and repeat the measurement
    c) Add more weight and repeat the measurement
    d) Switch to applanation tonometry

Chapter 7

Ocular
Pharmacology

1. **Anesthesia used to induce sleep is known as:**
   a) Topical anesthesia
   b) Regional anesthesia
   c) Local anesthesia
   d) General anesthesia

2. **An example of a procedure that would use local anesthetic is:**
   a) Cataract extraction on an infant
   b) Chalazion excision on an adult
   c) Noncontact tonometry
   d) Corneal topography studies

3. **Local anesthetic can be injected into the area of the nerve that supplies sensation to the surgical site. This is known as a:**
   a) Regional block
   b) Site-specific local
   c) General
   d) Topical

4. **The type of anesthesia named in the above question might be used for which surgical situation?**
   a) Chalazion excision
   b) Corneal transplant
   c) Radial keratotomy
   d) Laser trabeculoplasty

5. **Epinephrine might be added to a local anesthetic in order to:**
   a) Increase systemic absorption of the drug
   b) Reduce bleeding at the surgical site
   c) Enhance wound healing
   d) Move the anesthetic out of the area quickly

6. **Hyaluronidase is sometimes added to a local anesthetic in order to:**
   a) Reduce bleeding at the surgical site
   b) Increase systemic absorption of the drug
   c) Increase local spreading of the drug
   d) Decrease systemic absorption of the drug

7. **In addition to eliminating sensation, local anesthetic is sometimes required to:**
   a) Temporarily block vision
   b) Prevent movement
   c) Calm the patient
   d) Irrigate the surgical site

8. **Which of the following are commonly used local anesthetics?**
   a) Lidocaine, procaine
   b) Cocaine, proparacaine
   c) Butane, tetracaine
   d) Benoxinate, butacaine

9. **The most common side effect of local anesthetic is:**
   a) Cardiac arrest
   b) Respiratory arrest
   c) Increased blood pressure
   d) Dizziness and nausea

10. **Other side effects of local anesthetics include:**
    a) Lowered blood pressure, slowing of respiration
    b) Lowered blood pressure, rapid heartbeat
    c) Increased blood pressure, rapid respiration
    d) Increased blood pressure, respiratory collapse

11. **Which of the following drugs is an anesthetic?**
    a) Mannitol
    b) Cortisone
    c) Cocaine
    d) Betaxolol

12. **All of the following procedures are routinely performed after giving the patient topical anesthetic *except*:**
    a) Specular microscopy
    b) Pachymetry
    c) Initial contact lens fitting
    d) Applanation tonometry

13. **The most common side effect of topical anesthetics is:**
    a) Contact allergic reaction
    b) Fainting
    c) Increased blood pressure
    d) Dizziness

14. **Which of the following are commonly used topical anesthetics?**
    a) Cocaine, butacaine
    b) Proparacaine, tetracaine
    c) Procaine, lidocaine
    d) Prilocaine, epinephrine

15. **After instilling a topical anesthetic into the eye, the patient should be warned:**
    a) To keep the eyes dry
    b) To keep the eyes closed
    c) To be careful driving
    d) Not to rub the eye

16. **The function of mydriatics is to:**
    a) Decrease sensation and mobility
    b) Stimulate the dilator muscle of the iris
    c) Inhibit accommodation
    d) Lower intraocular pressure (IOP)

17. **During the routine eye exam, mydriatics are used to:**
    a) Facilitate applanation tonometry
    b) Facilitate examination of the fundus
    c) Facilitate refractometry
    d) Increase patient comfort

18. **The most common mydriatic in ophthalmic use is:**
    a) Tropicamide
    b) Epinephrine
    c) Cocaine
    d) Phenylephrine

19. **Phenylephrine causes dilation how quickly and wears off how quickly?**
    a) Dilation in 15 minutes, wears off in 1 to 2 hours
    b) Dilation in 15 minutes, wears off in 24 hours
    c) Dilation in 5 minutes, wears off in 30 minutes
    d) Dilation in 30 minutes, wears off in 5 to 6 hours

20. **The strength of phenylephrine that most commonly is used and is associated with fewer side effects is:**
    a) 0.1%
    b) 2.5%
    c) 10%
    d) 25%

21. **All of the following patient conditions call for cautious use of phenylephrine *except*:**
    a) Heart disease
    b) Some antidepressants
    c) Diabetes
    d) Hypertension

22. **The function of cycloplegics is to:**
    a) Decrease sensation and mobility of the eye
    b) Stimulate the dilator muscle of the iris
    c) Paralyze the ciliary muscle and sphincter muscles of the iris
    d) Paralyze the ciliary muscle and dilator muscle of the iris

23. **In ophthalmology, cycloplegics mainly are used to:**
    a) Facilitate corneal and retinal examination
    b) Facilitate iris photography
    c) Facilitate retinoscopy and refractometry
    d) Facilitate applanation tonometry

24. **Cycloplegic agents are used in the treatment of:**
    a) Presbyopia
    b) Iritis
    c) Retinitis pigmentosa
    d) Glaucoma

25. **Match the facts with the cycloplegic agent. (Agents may be used more than once.)**

A. The strongest drug	a) Atropine
B. Most rapid onset	b) Homatropine
C. Wears off in 10 to 14 days	c) Hyoscine
D. Wears off in 1 to 3 days	d) Cyclopentolate
E. Wears off in 1 hour	e) Tropicamide
F. Used three times daily for 3 days before exam	
G. Wears off in 3 to 6 hours	
H. Weak; used more for dilation	
I. Duration falls between atropine and homatropine	
J. Onset 30 minutes	

26. **Side effects caused by systemic absorption of a cycloplegic agent may be manifest by:**
    a) Increased pulse rate, flushing, fever, and dry mouth
    b) Decreased pulse rate, pallor, chills, and increased salivation
    c) Irregular pulse rate, cyanosis, chills, and sweating
    d) Flushing, rapid respiration, and increased salivation

27. **When one wishes to cycloplege a patient with dark eyes, it may be necessary to:**
    a) Use a topical anesthetic first
    b) Repeat doses or use stronger concentrations
    c) Use dilation reversal drops after the exam
    d) Delay refractometry until the drops have worn off

28. **Which of the following patients will be more difficult to dilate and/or cycloplege?**
    a) The patient using Propine
    b) The patient using pilocarpine
    c) The patient using a beta blocker
    d) The patient using a CAI

29. **Before instilling mydriatic or cycloplegic agents, it is most important to:**
    a) Check the patient's IOP
    b) Check the patient's pupillary response
    c) Check the patient's angles
    d) Check the patient's refractive error

30. **Which of the following tests would *not* give reliable results if performed after cycloplegia?**
    a) A scan for axial length
    b) Near point of convergence
    c) Tonometry
    d) Retinoscopy

31. **The most common side effect of mydriatics and cycloplegics is/are:**
    a) Stinging and contact allergy
    b) Lightheadedness and fainting
    c) Rapid respiration and heartbeat
    d) Nausea and vomiting

32. **Mydriatic and cycloplegic agents are identified by a:**
    a) Green top
    b) Red top
    c) Purple top
    d) Brown bottle

33. **Another name for epinephrine is:**
    a) Norepinephrine
    b) Acetylcholine
    c) Adrenaline
    d) Carbonic anhydrase

34. **The most common use of topical ocular medications containing epinephrine is:**
    a) Dilation
    b) Glaucoma treatment
    c) Decrease wound bleeding
    d) Dry eye treatment

35. **Many ophthalmologists and patients prefer epinephrine derivatives over miotics for glaucoma treatment because:**
    a) Epinephrine is available in gel form
    b) Miotics don't have to be instilled as often
    c) Epinephrine has fewer side effects
    d) Epinephrine lasts for 24 hours

36. **Which of the following glaucoma drops does *not* contain epinephrine?**
    a) Glaucon
    b) P1E1
    c) Iopidine
    d) Epinal

37. **The most commonly used epinephrine derivative is:**
    a) Betagan
    b) Timoptic
    c) Propine
    d) Pilopine

38. **Propine solution is marketed as:**
    a) 0.1%
    b) 0.5%
    c) 1.0%
    d) 5.0%

39. **Epinephrine stimulates the "fight or flight" (sympathetic) division of the nervous system. Therefore, its side effects may include:**
    a) Rapid pulse and respiration, stomach upset
    b) Muscle cramps, dry mouth
    c) Headache, accommodative spasms
    d) Slow pulse and respiration, increased digestion

40. **Epinephrine and epinephrine derivatives should be used with caution in patients with:**
    a) Rheumatoid arthritis, gout, and lupus
    b) Human Immunodeficiency Virus (HIV) and Herpes infections
    c) Cardiovascular disease, diabetes, and asthma
    d) Diverticulosis, stomach ulcers, and gastroenteritis

41. **Epinephrine and epinephrine derivatives generally are contraindicated in patients with:**
    a) Open-angle glaucoma
    b) Narrow angles
    c) IOL implants
    d) Hypertensive retinopathy

42. **Which of the following is *not* a beta blocker?**
    a) Timolol
    b) Soperonol
    c) Levobunolol
    d) Betaxolol

43. **Which of the following is *not* a beta blocker?**
    a) Ocupress
    b) Optipranolol
    c) Betagan
    d) Iopidine

44. **Beta blockers are identified by:**
    a) Purple caps
    b) Green or red caps
    c) Blue or yellow caps
    d) Brown bottles

45. **Which of the following is *not* true regarding beta blockers?**
    a) They can be used in addition to miotics and epinephrine compounds
    b) They act by reducing aqueous production
    c) They are safe to use even in cases of chronic obstructive pulmonary disease
    d) They are convenient because they usually are administered twice daily

46. **Before beginning a patient on a beta blocker for glaucoma, the physician may request:**
    a) Complete blood work
    b) A baseline blood pressure
    c) A chest X-ray
    d) Oxygen saturation

47. **The unique feature of the beta blocker Timoptic XE is:**
    a) It comes in unit dose capsules
    b) It is available over the counter
    c) It has the least side effects
    d) It forms a gel when applied

48. **Systemically, beta blockers are used to treat:**
    a) Congestive heart failure and hypertension
    b) Fluid retention and insomnia
    c) Asthma
    d) Inflammatory conditions

49. **Which of the following would have fewer side effects and be safer to use in a patient with a history of lung problems?**
    a) Timoptic
    b) Betagan
    c) Betoptic
    d) Optipranolol

50. **Possible side effects of beta blockers include:**
    a) Decreased heart rate and decreased respiration rate
    b) Decreased heart rate and increased respiration rate
    c) Increased heart and increased respiration rate
    d) Increased heart rate and decreased respiration rate

51. **Other side effects of beta blockers can include:**
    a) Miosis and ciliary spasms
    b) Depression, insomnia, and impotence
    c) Increased need of insulin in diabetics
    d) Depression of the immune system

52. **Miotics exert their effect by:**
    a) Stimulating the trabecular meshwork
    b) Stimulating the dilator muscle of the iris
    c) Stimulating the sphincter muscle of the iris
    d) Stimulating the ciliary body

53. **Miotics may be used in all of the following** *except*:
    a) Open and closed angle glaucoma
    b) Overcorrection following refractive surgery
    c) Convergent strabismus
    d) Posterior subcapsular cataracts

54. **Miotics act to lower IOP by:**
    a) Increasing aqueous outflow
    b) Decreasing aqueous production
    c) Providing a new outlet for aqueous drainage
    d) Dilating the pupil

55. **Which of the following is the most commonly used miotic for IOP control?**
    a) Carbachol
    b) Dapiprazole
    c) Echothiophate iodide
    d) Pilocarpine

56. **Which of the following is a miotic available in gel form for once a day use?**
    a) Carbachol
    b) Timolol
    c) Pilocarpine
    d) Dapiprazole

57. **Which of the following is part of the patient education information regarding use of miotics?**
    a) Call the office immediately if you experience headaches
    b) Discontinue the medication if you experience headaches
    c) Any drug-related headaches usually go away with continued use
    d) This medication frequently causes headaches during the entire time it is used

58. **Ocular side effects of miotics include all of the following** *except*:
    a) Spasms of the ciliary muscle
    b) Spasms of the sphincter muscle
    c) Local allergic reaction
    d) Decreased vision if cataracts are present
    d) Isoflurophate

59. **The systemic side effects most likely to occur in miotics include:**
    a) Decreased respiration, irregular heartbeat, and dry mouth
    b) Ciliary spasm, cataracts, and retinal detachment
    c) Increased blood pressure, excitability, and hallucinations
    d) Decreased blood pressure, cardiac arrest, sweating, and lethargy

60. **The main use of dapiprazole is:**
    a) IOP control
    b) Dilation reversal
    c) Amblyopia penalization
    d) Strabismus resolution

61. **Prior to use, patients should be told that dapiprazole will most likely:**
    a) Sting and cause redness
    b) Blur vision for an hour
    c) Change their eye color
    d) Cause IOP to rise

62. **The trade name for dapiprazole is:**
    a) Paremyd
    b) Phenoptic
    c) Rev-Eyes
    d) Carbastat

63. **Steroids are used to treat:**
    a) Bacterial infections
    b) Viral infections
    c) Inflammatory conditions
    d) Glaucoma

64. **All of the following would logically be treated with topical steroids *except*:**
    a) Iritis
    b) Scleritis and episcleritis
    c) Herpes zoster ophthalmicus
    d) Herpes simplex keratitis

65. **In ophthalmology, oral steroids are usually used in cases of:**
    a) Disorders involving the conjunctiva and cornea
    b) Secondary glaucoma
    c) Disorders involving the anterior segment
    d) Disorders involving the posterior segment

66. **All of the following are examples of steroids *except*:**
    a) Prednisolone
    b) Diazepam
    c) Dexamethasone
    d) Hydrocortisone

67. **Which of the following are topical steroid drops?**
    a) Inflamase Forte, FML, Pred Forte
    b) Blephamide, Cortisporin, Maxitrol, TobraDex
    c) Ocufen, Voltaren, Acular PF
    d) Tobrex, Genoptic, Ciloxin

68. **Your patient has been taking topical steroids four times a day for iritis. There are no longer signs of inflammation in the anterior chamber. Most likely the physician will have the patient:**
    a) Stop the medication
    b) Increase the drops to six times a day
    c) Gradually decrease the drops
    d) Switch to an antibiotic to ward off secondary infection

69. **Your patient is taking topical steroid drops for keratitis. Which of the following tests is most important?**
    a) Applanation tonometry
    b) Color vision test
    c) Glare test
    d) Corneal topography

70. **Your patient is taking oral steroids for posterior uveitis. Which of the following tests or exams is most important?**
    a) Fundus exam
    b) Slit lamp exam
    c) Schirmer's tear test
    d) Extraocular muscle function tests

71. **The systemic side effects of steroids include:**
    a) Dizziness, dehydration, elevated blood pressure, and insomnia
    b) Headaches, sleeplessness, hallucinations, and increased pulse
    c) Dehydration, lowered blood pressure, excitability, and confusion
    d) Sweating, elevated blood pressure, weakness, and delayed wound healing

72. **A serious drawback of oral or topical steroids is that they can:**
    a) Boost the immune system
    b) Depress the immune system
    c) Cause strokes
    d) Decrease blood glucose levels

73. **Ocular side effects of topical steroids can include:**
    a) Development of subcapsular cataracts
    b) Subnormal IOP
    c) Miotic pupil
    d) Accommodative spasms

74. **Topical steroids are frequently combined with which of the following?**
    a) Epinephrine to lower IOP
    b) NSAIDs to decrease inflammation
    c) Antivirals to combat infection
    d) Antibiotics to combat infection

75. **Antibiotics are used in ophthalmology in cases of:**
    a) Fungal infections
    b) Bacterial infections
    c) Viral infections
    d) Allergic reactions

76. **Antibiotics that kill microorganisms are called:**
    a) Sulfonamides
    b) Bacteriocidal
    c) Bacteriostatic
    d) Antiseptics

77. **Antibiotics that inhibit the reproduction and growth of microorganisms are called:**
    a) Penicillins
    b) Bacteriocidal
    c) Bacteriostatic
    d) Germicidal

78. **Bacteriocidal antibiotics include:**
    a) Tetracycline and erythromycin
    b) Penicillin, streptomycin, and ampicillin
    c) Sulfisoxazole and sodium sulfacetamide
    d) Acyclovir, idoxuridine, and trifluridine

79. **Bacteriostatic antibiotics include:**
    a) Genoptic, Cetamide, and Tobrex
    b) Vitrasert, Herplex, and Viroptic
    c) Refresh, Lacrilube, and Murine
    d) Ak-Sulf, Bleph 10, and Isopto Cetamide

80. **In order to select an antibiotic that will kill a specific microorganism, the physician might order:**
    a) A biopsy
    b) A slit lamp exam
    c) A culture
    d) A fluorescein angiogram

81. **An antibiotic that will kill many different types of microorganisms would be referred to as:**
    a) Broad spectrum
    b) Narrow spectrum
    c) Bacteriostatic
    d) Hypereffective

82. **What should patients be told regarding the use of oral antibiotics?**
    a) Take it until you feel better, then discontinue
    b) Take several days' worth, then discontinue even if you have medication left
    c) Take all but 2 days' worth, in order to save some in case you relapse later
    d) Take all of the medication until it's gone, even if you feel well

83. **Which topical antibiotic is most likely to cause a local allergic reaction?**
    a) Tobramycin
    b) Gentamicin
    c) Neomycin
    d) Erythromycin

84. **Which topical antibiotic is most likely to cause a local reaction?**
    a) Tobrex
    b) Genoptic
    c) AK-Sulf
    d) Romycin

85. **Systemic effects of antibiotics, especially oral antibiotics, can include all of the following *except*:**
    a) Development of resistant bacteria
    b) Allergic and anaphylactic reactions
    c) Gastrointestinal disturbance
    d) Increased blood glucose levels

86. **What percentage of the population is reported to be allergic to penicillin?**
    a) 10%
    b) 15%
    c) 20%
    d) 30%

87. **CAIs have what effect on the eye?**
    a) Reduce corneal edema
    b) Lower IOP
    c) Stimulate accommodation
    d) Reduce inflammation

88. **CAIs are used in the treatment of glaucoma because they:**
    a) Increase aqueous outflow
    b) Decrease aqueous outflow
    c) Increase aqueous production
    d) Reduce aqueous production

89. **The generic name for Diamox is:**
    a) Mannitol
    b) Methazolamide
    c) Acetazolamide
    d) Dichlorphenamide

90. **Diamox is available as:**
    a) 500 mg sequels
    b) 50 mg tablets
    c) Vials for home injection
    d) 2% ophthalmic solution

91. **All of the following are topical medications containing CAIs for glaucoma treatment except:**
    a) Lumigan
    b) Trusopt
    c) Azopt
    d) CoSopt

92. **The most common side effect of oral CAIs is:**
    a) Development of kidney stones
    b) Tingling of the extremities
    c) Metallic taste in the mouth
    d) Depression and fatigue

93. **CAIs should not be given to patients who are allergic to:**
    a) Penicillin
    b) Sulfa drugs
    c) Sulfur drugs
    d) Erythromycin

94. **Vasoconstrictors act by:**
    a) Constricting blood vessels
    b) Constricting the heart
    c) Constricting the dilator muscle
    d) Constricting the crystalline lens

95. **Vasoconstrictors are used to:**
    a) Lower IOP
    b) Enhance drug absorption
    c) "Whiten" the eye
    d) Reduce itching and watering

96. **Vasoconstrictors also are known by the term:**
    a) Antibiotics
    b) Antihistamines
    c) Decongestants
    d) Lubricators

97. Which of the following is *not* commonly used as a decongestant?
    a) Phenylephrine
    b) Scopolamine
    c) Tetrahydrozoline
    d) Naphazoline

98. Use of vasoconstrictors is contraindicated in the patient with:
    a) Dry eye
    b) Hay fever
    c) Subconjunctival hemorrhage
    d) Tired, red eyes

99. The purpose of antihistamines is to block the release of histamine, thus:
    a) Lowering IOP
    b) Reversing pupil dilation
    c) Blocking some symptoms of the allergic response
    d) Stopping the allergic response

100. All of the following are topical antihistamines *except*:
    a) Elestat
    b) Naphcon A
    c) Opticrom
    d) Patanol

101. Topical antihistamines are combined frequently with:
    a) Antivirals
    b) Decongestants
    c) Steroids
    d) Nonsteroidal anti-inflammatories

102. All of the following are *false* regarding antihistamines *except*:
    a) They are available only by prescription
    b) Topical preparations have no systemic side effects
    c) Some oral preparations may cause drowsiness
    d) They are used to treat infection

103. Oral and intravenous osmotics are used in the treatment of:
    a) Corneal edema
    b) Angle-closure glaucoma
    c) Open-angle glaucoma
    d) Iritis

104. Osmotics exert their effect by:
    a) Drawing water out of the tissues
    b) Drawing water out of the blood stream
    c) Causing blood vessels to constrict
    d) Causing blood vessels to dilate

105. Oral glycerin and isosorbide are best administered:
    a) Diluted with water
    b) Straight from the bottle so it can be drunk quickly
    c) Followed by 32 ounces of water
    d) Over ice and sipped slowly with a straw

106. **Which is an oral osmotic that would be safer for a diabetic patient?**
    a) Ismotic
    b) Osmoglyn
    c) Glyrol
    d) Mannitol

107. **Which of the following are osmotics available for intravenous use?**
    a) Glycerin and isosorbide
    b) Osmitrol and glycerol
    c) Sucrose and lactose
    d) Mannitol and urea

108. **If a patient who is being given an oral osmotic for rapid IOP reduction complains of thirst, she should:**
    a) Be given more osmotic
    b) Be given a drink of water
    c) Not be given anything to drink
    d) Be told to lie down

109. **Other side effects of oral or IV osmotics include:**
    a) Lacrimation, excess salivation, and insomnia
    b) Dehydration, headache, and disorientation
    c) Tissue edema, metallic taste, and tingling of extremities
    d) Ringing in the ears, kidney stones, and back pain

110. **Topical osmotics work by:**
    a) Creating a low osmotic pressure in the tears, drawing fluid out of the cornea
    b) Creating a high osmotic pressure in the tears, drawing fluid out of the cornea
    c) Creating a low osmotic pressure in the cornea, causing fluid to filter out
    d) Creating a high osmotic pressure in the tears, forcing fluid into the cornea

111. **A commonly used topical osmotic for the long-term treatment of corneal edema is:**
    a) Mannitol
    b) Rose bengal
    c) Sodium chloride drops or ointment
    d) Fluorescein sodium solution

112. **An in-office use of topical anhydrous glycerin is:**
    a) Quick lowering of IOP
    b) Temporary corneal clearing for examination purposes
    c) Enhancing dilation for examination purposes
    d) Reversing dilation

113. **A disadvantage to use of topical osmotic agents is:**
    a) Ocular discomfort
    b) Ciliary spasm
    c) Brow ache
    d) Blurred vision

114. **Topical nonsteroidal anti-inflammatory drugs (NSAIDs) are indicated in all of the following *except*:**
    a) Reducing postoperative inflammation
    b) Elimination of most ocular allergic symptoms
    c) Relief of allergic itching
    d) Preventing pupillary miosis during surgery

115. NSAIDs act by:
   a) Blocking the release of histamine
   b) Stimulating the dilator muscle
   c) Blocking the release of prostaglandins
   d) Drawing fluid out of the tissues

116. Topical NSAIDs are sometimes preferred over steroids because:
   a) They do not significantly elevate IOP with long-term use
   b) They control inflammation better
   c) They can be combined with antibiotics
   d) They do not sting on instillation

117. All of the following are topical NSAIDs *except*:
   a) Ocufen
   b) FML
   c) Voltaren
   d) Acular PF

118. In which situation is use of topical NSAIDs contraindicated?
   a) Mild uveitis
   b) Acute infection
   c) Postoperative refractive surgery
   d) Allergic conjunctivitis

119. Match the medication with its type/purpose (an answer may be used more than once).

Iopidine	a) Antiviral
Refresh	b) Antifungal
Tensilon	c) Diagnostic stain/dye
Healon	d) Tears and lubricants
Polysporin	e) Used in evaluating ptosis
Lacrilube	f) Used to lower IOP after laser treatment
Celluvisc	g) Steroid antibiotic combination
Ocuvite	h) Antibiotic combination
Viscoat	i) Vitamins formulated for ocular health
Ciloxan	j) Lens coupling agent
rose bengal	k) Viscoelastic agent
Viroptic	l) Treatment of macular degeneration
Gonak	
Lacrisert	
TobraDex	
fluorescein	
Maxitrol	
Quixin	
Neosporin	
Hypotears	
Macugen	
trypan blue	
Goniosol	
Ocucaps	
acyclovir	
Natacyn	
Enlon	

120. **Your patient may have a corneal abrasion, so you have instilled topical fluorescein. What else must you do to view the cornea most clearly?**
    a) Use a cobalt blue light
    b) Use an ultraviolet light
    c) Use polarized light
    d) Use a red-free light

121. **In which condition would using rose bengal be of most benefit?**
    a) Glaucoma
    b) Severe dry eye
    c) Conjunctival injection
    d) Corneal foreign body

122. **Vidarabine is used specifically to treat:**
    a) Herpes zoster
    b) Herpes simplex
    c) Bacterial conjunctivitis with allergic response
    d) Lice living on the lash line

123. **Vitamins and minerals that have been indicated in treatment of macular degeneration are:**
    a) Vitamins B, B_{12}, D, and magnesium
    b) Vitamin C, calcium, and iron
    c) Vitamin D, fluoride, and manganese
    d) Vitamins A, C, E, and zinc

124. **Patients who use nonpreserved artificial tears supplied in "bullets" should be told to:**
    a) Use them only once a day
    b) Discard the leftover solution at the end of the day
    c) Use them only at night
    d) Make their own saline because it's cheaper

125. **Dry eye patients should be told to use artificial tears:**
    a) Morning and night
    b) Only when the eyes water
    c) Four times daily
    d) As often as needed to control symptoms

126. **An injection of edrophonium chloride (Tensilon) is used to:**
    a) Determine if a ptosis is due to myasthenia gravis
    b) Determine if a ptosis is due to congenital defect
    c) Determine if a ptosis is due to a levator weakness
    d) Identify Horner's syndrome

127. **Botulinum toxin injection is used to relieve:**
    a) Accommodative esotropia
    b) Accommodative spasms
    c) Blepharospasms
    d) Migraine headaches

128. **In ophthalmology, prostaglandin analogues are used to treat:**
    a) Glaucoma
    b) Allergy symptoms
    c) Infection
    d) Inflammation

129. **Topical ophthalmic alpha-2 agonists are used to:**
    a) Reduce inflammation
    b) Lower IOP
    c) Treat ocular symptoms of AIDS
    d) Reduce allergy symptoms

130. **The best pH (acid/alkaline) for topical eye medications is:**
    a) Between 3 and 4
    b) Between 6 and 8
    c) Between 9 and 10
    d) Between 11 and 12

131. **Agents that may be added to most any ophthalmic drug preparation include:**
    a) Buffers, preservatives, vehicles, chelating agents
    b) Ointments, drops, gels, strips, and sprays
    c) Miotics, cycloplegics, and mydriatics
    d) Epinephrine, hyaluronidase, and tetrahydroziline

132. **The most ideal drug for treatment of chronic open-angle glaucoma:**
    a) Effectively lowers IOP
    b) Has no side effects
    c) Requires once-a-day dosing
    d) All of the above

133. **Which of the following is recommended to minimize the systemic absorption of a topical ophthalmic medication?**
    a) Dilute the medication with artificial tears
    b) Close eyes and press on the nasolacrimal area
    c) Use ointment rather than drops
    d) Decrease the dosing frequency by half

Chapter 8

Photography

1. **Every camera includes the following elements:**
   a) Aperture, shutter, and film
   b) Lens, film, and diaphragm
   c) Camera body, lens, and frame counter
   d) Aperture, camera body, and film

2. **A good camera lens system will:**
   a) Effectively focus an image at any distance from the subject
   b) Have the same focal length for all film formats
   c) Be made up of only plus (convex) lenses
   d) Produce sharp images on the film plane when properly focused

3. **All films, black and white or color:**
   a) Are sensitive to some form of light
   b) Produce equally sharp images
   c) Have similarly sized silver grains
   d) Can be used for ophthalmic photography

4. **Film speed refers to:**
   a) How quickly it can be processed
   b) Its ability to photograph moving subjects
   c) Its sensitivity to light
   d) The length of time required to expose the film

5. **Which of the following films is most sensitive?**
   a) 25 ISO
   b) 400 ISO
   c) Negative transparency
   d) Print film

6. **A slower film will have:**
   a) A low ISO number, finer grains, and better resolution
   b) A high ISO number, coarser grains, and better resolution
   c) A low ISO number, coarser grains, and better resolution
   d) A low ISO number, finer grains, and poorer resolution

7. **For the most part, a faster film will have:**
   a) A sharper image quality
   b) A poorer image quality
   c) A longer exposure time
   d) A shorter developing time

8. **The image produced on color slide film:**
   a) Is a negative image
   b) Is a positive image
   c) Is produced from negatives
   d) Is less sharp than prints

9. **The size of the silver particles in the film emulsion is referred to as:**
   a) Density
   b) Grain
   c) Contrast index
   d) Sensitivity

10. **The capability of a film to produce variations of highlights and shadows is the:**
    a) Film speed
    b) Exposure
    c) Film density
    d) Contrast index

11. **Film exposure is directly related to:**
    a) The length of time that the film is in the developing solution
    b) The length of time that the light strikes the film
    c) The saturation of chemicals of the developing solution
    d) The focal length of the lens system

12. **Film exposure is controlled by:**
    a) The strength of the chemicals in the developing solution
    b) The length of time that the film is left in the developing solution
    c) Proper focusing of the lens system
    d) Shutter speed, film sensitivity, and f-stop

13. **Each higher f-stop setting and each lower shutter speed setting increases film exposure:**
    a) By 25%
    b) By a factor of two
    c) By a factor of 10
    d) By one log unit

14. **A shutter setting of 30 means that the film is exposed for:**
    a) 30 seconds
    b) 3.00 seconds
    c) 0.30 seconds
    d) 1/30 of a second

15. **At which f-stop setting would the most light be allowed to reach the film?**
    a) 0
    b) 1
    c) 8
    d) 32

16. **If the f-stop and/or shutter speed is off by so much as one setting, the film may be:**
    a) Over- or underexposed
    b) Unexposed
    c) Unprocessable
    d) Double exposed

17. **The focal length of a camera lens is defined as:**
    a) The distance between the film and the subject
    b) The distance between the lens and the subject
    c) The distance between the lens and the film
    d) The distance between the lens and the object in focus

18. **Which of the following lenses makes the image appear larger or closer because of its longer focal length?**
    a) Telephoto
    b) Normal
    c) Wide-angle
    d) Micro lens

19. **Which of the following lenses has a variable focal length?**
    a) Soper lens
    b) Macro lens
    c) Zoom lens
    d) Micro lens

20. **Depth of field is defined as:**
    a) The point at which the camera is focused
    b) The distance between the subject and the film
    c) The distance range within which objects are focused clearly
    d) The width of the field that will appear on the film

21. **As a general rule, the depth of field covers:**
    a) A field width equal to 1/2 of that of the human eye
    b) The entire field visible through the camera
    c) 1/2 behind and 1/2 in front of the point of focus
    d) 2/3 behind and 1/3 in front of the point of focus

22. **The larger the f-stop number:**
    a) The smaller the depth of field
    b) The larger the depth of field
    c) The wider the depth of field
    d) The more resolution in the photograph

23. **At an f-stop setting of 16, which lens will give the greater depth of field?**
    a) Wide-angle lens
    b) Telephoto lens
    c) Standard 50 mm lens
    d) Long focal length

24. **In addition to being affected by f-stop and focal length, depth of field depends on:**
    a) Film speed
    b) Whether the film is color or black and white
    c) Distance from camera to subject
    d) Shutter speed

25. **A deeper depth of field will result directly from all of the following *except*:**
    a) A lens with a short focal length
    b) A larger f-stop setting
    c) A faster shutter speed
    d) A longer camera-to-subject distance

26. **The term *synchronization* means that:**
    a) The shutter is fully opened at the same time that available light is at maximum
    b) The shutter is fully opened at the same time the flash illumination is at maximum
    c) The f-stop and shutter speed are set appropriately to match the film speed
    d) The focal length and camera-to-subject distance are coordinated

27. **If the synchronization connector is not attached properly, the resulting photographs may be:**
    a) Exposed only on one side
    b) Overexposed
    c) Underexposed
    d) Blurred

28. **In a camera with an electronic flash, the synchronization cord should be connected to the:**
   a) FP outlet on the camera
   b) X outlet on the camera
   c) M outlet on the camera
   d) KH outlet on the camera

29. **In order to produce two images, the beam splitter utilizes:**
   a) Prisms
   b) Mirrors
   c) Lenses
   d) Filters

30. **A beam splitter is necessary on a slit lamp camera in order to:**
   a) Produce an image for each ocular
   b) Reduce the illumination in the oculars
   c) Increase the illumination
   d) Produce an image in the oculars and in the camera

31. **The main problem with beam splitters is that:**
   a) Only low levels of illumination can be used
   b) Less light reaches the oculars, reducing detail
   c) Less light reaches the subject, reducing detail
   d) They must be flipped out of the way when taking a photograph

32. **In fundus photography, in order to achieve a clear image at the film plane:**
   a) The reticule and subject must be in focus simultaneously
   b) The ocular(s) must be set for the subject's refractive error
   c) The diopter correction dial must be set at plus
   d) The ocular(s) must be set at zero

33. **The reticule is designed to be focused at:**
   a) The film plane
   b) The focal length of the lens
   c) Infinity
   d) The distance from the subject

34. **The purpose of the reticule in fundus photography is:**
   a) To compensate for the subject's refractive error
   b) To compensate for the photographer's refractive error
   c) To superimpose a measurement scale on each photograph
   d) To provide a reference point for focusing

35. **Setting the fundus camera eyepiece should be done:**
   a) With one eye shut, in dim light or darkness
   b) With both eyes open, in dim light or darkness
   c) With both eyes open in a normally lit room
   d) With one eye shut in a normally lit room

36. **When setting the ocular of the fundus camera system, one must:**
   a) Remove one's own correction
   b) Turn the ocular to the maximum plus position, then rotate down
   c) Turn the ocular to the maximum plus position, then rotate up
   d) Turn the ocular to the maximum minus position, then rotate up

37. **If you continue to turn the ocular past the first point of clarity:**
    a) The reticule will become sharper yet
    b) You can compensate for the patient's refractive error
    c) You may induce your own accommodation
    d) The resulting photograph will be sharper

38. **In fundus photography:**
    a) The clarity of the cornea and lens do not make a difference in photo clarity
    b) The camera's internal lens system is the only consideration
    c) The patient's cornea and lens become part of the camera's optical system
    d) The dioptric power of the lens and cornea are discounted

39. **If the image seems to go in and out of focus, yet the fundus camera and patient are held stationary:**
    a) The photographer probably is accommodating
    b) The patient probably is blinking
    c) The patient is not fixating properly
    d) The patient has fatigued

40. **You are attempting to take fundus photographs, and see a blue-gray halo around the subject. To correct this, you should:**
    a) Move the camera closer
    b) Move the camera farther back
    c) Reduce illumination
    d) Increase illumination

41. **You are attempting to take fundus photographs and notice a whitish haze in the center of the subject. This may mean that:**
    a) The patient is highly myopic
    b) The patient is highly hyperopic
    c) The patient has his eye closed
    d) The camera has drifted forward

42. **Gross focusing with the fundus camera is generally accomplished by:**
    a) Turning the eyepiece until the subject is clear
    b) Moving the joy stick
    c) Having the patient lean forward or back
    d) Changing the magnification setting

43. **Focusing the fundus camera can be simplified by:**
    a) Starting with the camera all the way back, then moving it forward
    b) Starting with the camera all the way forward, then moving it back
    c) Focusing the donut on the patient's closed lid before composing the photograph
    d) Positioning the fixation light directly in front of the camera lens

44. **The main disadvantage of video recording is:**
    a) Expense of the equipment
    b) Poor resolution of the image
    c) Complexity of the equipment
    d) Difficulty in reproducing the film

45. **Uses of video systems in ophthalmology include all of the following *except*:**
    a) Specular microscopy
    b) Pachymetry
    c) Documenting surgical procedures
    d) Documenting eye movements (positions of gaze)

46. **Astigmatism during fundus photography may be induced by:**
    a) The patient's accommodation
    b) The photographer's accommodation
    c) The angle of the camera to the cornea
    d) Use of dioptric compensation

47. **The photographic result of uncorrected induced astigmatism is:**
    a) Overexposure
    b) A bright crescent at the periphery
    c) Blurring in one meridian
    d) Distortion

48. **Induced astigmatism or high corneal astigmatism can be compensated for by:**
    a) Use of the correction device in the fundus camera
    b) Placing the dioptric correction dial on "+" for plus cylinder
    c) Placing the dioptric correction dial on "−" for minus cylinder
    d) Having the patient wear a toric contact lens during photography

49. **The most important thing to do before using any fundus camera each day should be:**
    a) Confirm the diopter compensator is at the "+" setting
    b) Insure all patients are dilated with homatropine
    c) Check to see that the eyepiece reticule is correctly set
    d) Clean the camera lens whether or not it is dirty

50. **Proper pupil dilation to facilitate fundus photography requires:**
    a) Any dilation is acceptable
    b) Dilation is not necessary
    c) A minimum pupil size of 4 to 5 mm
    d) A minimum pupil size of 8 mm

51. **Always include all of the following techniques when performing fundus photography *except*:**
    a) Insure the camera is loaded with film
    b) Check the reticule setting on the fundus camera
    c) Explain the procedure to the patient
    d) Avoid all conversation once the patient is in position

52. **To allow scanning of the patient's retina without moving the base of the camera mount:**
    a) Move the fixation light and ask the patient to follow it
    b) Use the joy stick
    c) Adjust the chin cup
    d) Swing the camera on its pivot

53. **The primary component of the optical imaging system of the fundus camera:**
    a) Is an aspheric lens that acts as an indirect ophthalmoscope
    b) Is an astigmatic lens that acts as an indirect ophthalmoscope
    c) Is an aspheric lens that acts as a retinoscope
    d) Is a divergent lens that acts as a microscope

54. **The illumination exposure system of the fundus camera includes:**
    a) Both halogen and tungsten light bulbs
    b) A fixation light and flash system
    c) The view lamp and the electronic flash system
    d) A beam splitter and view lamp

55. **In order to view eyes with high refractive errors, it is best to:**
    a) Place a contact lens on the patient's eye to compensate
    b) Reset the eyepiece reticule to compensate
    c) Set the diopter compensation device built into the camera
    d) Eyes with high refractive errors cannot be photographed

56. **Before taking the fundus photograph, it is important to do all of the following** *except*:
    a) Check the patient's record to confirm the requested photographs
    b) Enter patient information into a log manual or camera imprint system
    c) Study any previous fundus photos that the patient has had
    d) Make sure that the patient has had a visual field test

57. **To take a photo of the external eye with the fundus camera (for example, to document corneal edema that interferes with a clear view of the fundus):**
    a) Change the diopter setting to "–"
    b) Change the diopter setting to "+"
    c) Have the patient sit back from the camera
    d) A slit lamp camera must be used

58. **When aligning the fundus camera, it is best to:**
    a) Have the patient look straight ahead while you look through the camera, adjusting the joy stick
    b) Have the patient close both eyes so you can see the donut projected on the eyelid as you adjust camera position
    c) Have the patient look straight ahead so you can see the donut projected on the cornea as you adjust camera position
    d) Have the patient sit back and relax until you have the camera in position

59. **When correctly positioned, the orange-yellow background of the fundus should be:**
    a) At an even color saturation across the viewing field
    b) Darker in the periphery of the viewing field
    c) Lighter in the periphery of the viewing field
    d) Unevenly saturated across the viewing field

60. **Once the fundal image is correctly positioned and focused:**
    a) Fire the camera
    b) Ask the patient to blink, then fire the camera
    c) Have the patient sit back and rest a moment
    d) Take repeated photographs quickly, warning the patient not to blink

61. **Periodic photographs to monitor the progress of a disease might be needed in all of the following** *except*:
    a) Active histoplasmosis scar
    b) Aphakia
    c) Diabetic retinopathy
    d) Glaucoma

62. **The primary area of interest in the fundus photo of a glaucoma patient is:**
    a) The optic disc
    b) The macula
    c) The retinal vessels
    d) The choroid

63. **In a diabetic survey, a series of photos are taken that include:**
    a) Five overlapping fields of view
    b) Four fields of view to document every quadrant
    c) Seven overlapping fields of view
    d) Two photos: one centered on the disc and one centered on the macula

64. **If the patient is to have fundus photos of both eyes:**
    a) Go from right eye to left eye without stopping to avoid patient fatigue
    b) Wait 30 minutes between photographing the right and left eye
    c) Allow the patient to rest in between until the fixation light can be seen
    d) Use stronger dilating drops on the second eye

65. **You are centering on the fundus when a light yellow crescent appears in the upper left of the viewing field. This is caused by:**
    a) Illumination set too high
    b) Reflection off of a cataract
    c) Pathology in the fundus
    d) Reflection off of the edge of the pupil

66. **In the scenario above, you should:**
    a) Reduce illumination
    b) Move the camera slightly down and to the right
    c) Move the camera slightly up and to the left
    d) Use the dioptric compensation device

67. **Poor detail on a fundus photograph can be caused by all of the following *except*:**
    a) Improper focusing
    b) Hazy media
    c) Retinal pathology
    d) Failing to set the eyepiece accurately

68. **Inadequate dilation results in photographs with:**
    a) Half of the frame unexposed
    b) A general blur
    c) A gray, fuzzy quadrant
    d) A grainy appearance

69. Matching. Match the artifact/error to the photograph (Figures 8-1 through 8-6):

A. Camera too close	a) Figure 8-1
B. Camera too far back	b) Figure 8-2
C. Film not completely advanced	c) Figure 8-3
D. Flash not synchronized with shutter	d) Figure 8-4
E. Patient blinked	e) Figure 8-5
F. Pupil cut	f) Figure 8-6

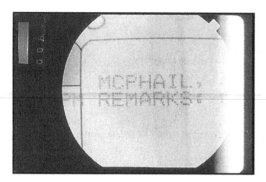

Figure 8-1. Photo courtesy of Eyesight Associates of Middle Georgia.

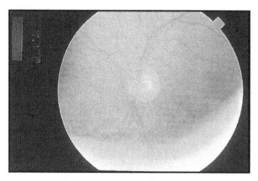

Figure 8-2. Photo courtesy of Eyesight Associates of Middle Georgia.

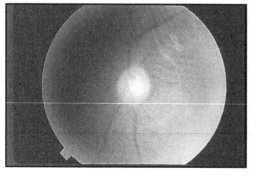

Figure 8-3. Photo courtesy of Eyesight Associates of Middle Georgia.

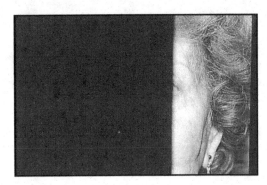

Figure 8-4. Photo courtesy of Eyesight Associates of Middle Georgia.

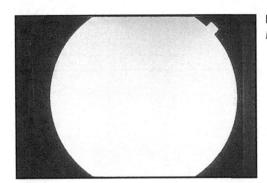

Figure 8-5. Photo courtesy of Eyesight Associates of Middle Georgia.

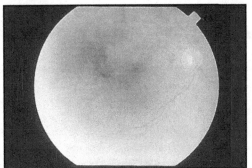

Figure 8-6. Photo courtesy of Eyesight Associates of Middle Georgia.

Chapter 9

Explanatory
Answers

Chapter 2. Clinical Optics

1. b) Depending on which reference is consulted, visible light is in the range of 400 to 800 nanometers. (Be sure to watch the units of measurement given in an answer. "Meters" in answer *d* should have indicated that it was incorrect.)

2. a) Infrared light borders the visible color red and ultraviolet light borders the visible color violet. All of the other answers are invisible components of the electromagnetic spectrum, but do not abut red or violet.

3. a) Red has the longest wavelength: 650 nanometers.

4. b) Geometric optics involves the reaction of light as it passes through media (any transparent object) or strikes a surface. Answers *a* and *d* refer to physical optics. Physiologic optics defines answer *c*.

5. a) When light strikes an object or an interface between media with different indices of refraction and bounces back, this is called *reflection*.

6. a) The light that hits the object or interface is termed *incident*. Those rays that bounce back from the object or interface are called *reflected*.

7. d) A medium is a transparent object through which light can pass. It is not a light source (ie, does not emit light). It does not necessarily refract light, either (see next question).

8. b) The quality of a medium to bend light is called *refraction*. In reflection, the rays are bounced off of the surface. Absorbed light does not pass through a medium. Tropism actually refers to the phenomenon of plants bending toward a light source.

9. a) The incident ray is the ray that first strikes and enters a medium. A divergent ray has been refracted outward. The emergent ray is the ray as it exits the medium. A parallel ray is straight.

10. d) If the light is spread apart by the lens, the rays are said to be divergent.

11. b) Convergence occurs when light rays are brought together (bent inward) by the lens.

12. a) The IR of a substance is found by dividing the speed of light in air by the speed of light through the substance. This is known as Snell's Law.

13. b) A substance with a high IR is more dense, and slows down the light passing through it.

14. d) Depending on which reference is consulted, the IR of crown glass is 1.50. Light traveling through a vacuum is zero, through air is 1.0, and through water is 1.33.

15. b) Light traveling through a prism is bent toward the prism's base.

16. d) Because light is bent toward the base, the image appears to be shifted toward the apex. A real image can be projected on a screen, while a virtual image cannot.

17. c) A 1.00 diopter prism bends light 1 cm at a distance of 1 m from the prism.

18. b) The formula for figuring prism displacement is P + C/D, where P is the prism power, C is the displacement of the object in cm, and D is the distance from the prism in meters. To plug in this problem: 2 = 1/D. Do algebra and multiply both sides by D/1, yielding 2D = 1. Now divide both sides by 2: D = 1/2. 1/2 equals 0.5 m.

19. d) Plug in again: P = 5/1. Thus P = 5.0 diopters.

20. c) Plug in to get: 12 = C/2. Multiply each side by 2/1, and 24 = C. The answer is 24 cm. (Be sure to pay attention to units of measurement! Another correct answer would have been 0.24 m.)

21. c) A spherical lens refracts light equally in every direction. This is evidenced by the fact that you can shine a light through a plus lens and focus it to a point.

22. b) A 1.00 diopter lens focuses light at 1 m. (Technically, the light entering the lens must be parallel for this to hold true.)

23. d) The focal point is the place where the lens focuses incoming light. The focal point may be real (can be projected onto a screen) or virtual (exists in theory but cannot be projected).

24. a) The optical center does not always coincide with the geometrical center of a lens. (The word "always" should have indicated that this answer was false.)

25. a) Measure the distance between the lens and the focal point, and you will have measured the focal length. It is related to the dioptric power of the lens in that the stronger the lens, the shorter the focal length.

26. b) The focal length of a minus lens exists in theory, so it *can* be calculated. But it is theoretical, in this case as virtual as the focal point.

27. c) The formula for focal length is P = 1/F. Answer *a* is the formula for IR, *b* is for prism displacement, and *d* is for finding the vergence of light rays.

28. d) P is 5 diopters. 5 = 1/F. Multiply each side by F/1, and get 5F = 1. Now divide each side by 5, and get F = 1/5 = 0.2 meters.

29. c) This time it's done backwards. F is 33 cm. The formula calls for meters, so change cm to m before doing the math. There are 100 cm in a meter, so 33 cm = 0.33 m. F is 0.33. Now plug into the formula: P = 1/0.33. Simple math, and you end up with 3.0 diopters.

30. Matching:

A. Virtual image	b
B. Converges light	a
C. Used to correct presbyopia in the emmetrope	a
D. Minifies	b
E. Barrel distortion	b
F. Concave	b
G. Thicker in the middle	a
H. Used to correct aphakia	a
I. Magnifies	a
J. Used to correct myopia	b
K. Two prisms placed base to base	a
L. Diverges light	b
M. Pincushion distortion	a
N. Used to correct hyperopia	a
O. Convex	a
P. Two prisms placed apex to apex	b
Q. Thinner in the middle	b
R. Real image	a

31. d) Cylindrical lenses can be plus or minus power.

32. c) The line of light projected by a lens lines up with the axis. To prove it, get the strongest plus cylinder lens you have in your trial set. Shine a pen light through it onto the wall. Move the lens and light back and forth a bit until the line focuses.

Figure 9-1. Conoid of Sturm formed by a spherocylindrical lens. Reprinted with permission from Lens A. *Optics, Retinoscopy, and Refractometry.* Thorofare, NJ: SLACK Incorporated; 1999.

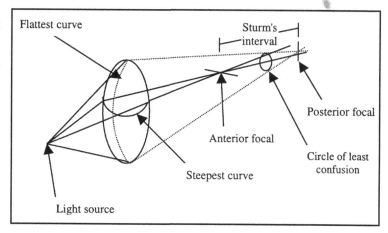

33. b) Between the anterior focal line and the posterior focal line is an area known as Sturm's interval.

34. d) The light rays in Sturm's interval are arranged in a cone-shape, and are called Sturm's conoid or the Conoid of Sturm (Figure 9-1).

35. a) The circle of least confusion is at the midpoint between the two focal lines of a spherocylindrical lens. While the image is not perfectly focused here, it is the most clear image available. The goal in using a cylinder to correct astigmatism is to collapse the Conoid of Sturm and place both focal lines on the retina, which gives a sharper focus than that at the circle of least confusion.

36. d) An optical cross is a way of diagramming the power of a lens in the two principle meridians (which are always 90 degrees from each other). *Note:* Some confusion has arisen in the past regarding the optical cross. The *true* optical cross is a representation of the effective power of a lens system. That is what is being discussed here. However, some clinicians use a cross to represent the patient's refractive error as measured on the phoropter. In this case, the power readings are taken right off the phoropter, representing the meridians where the patient's refractive error was neutralized, *not* where the lens system's effective power lies.

37. a) Since the power in each meridian is the same, this is a spherical lens of +3.00 power.

38. d) Remember this rule: whatever meridian you choose to start with when figuring the power, that also is going to be the axis of the answer. In this example, start with the zero (Plano). It is in the 90 degree meridian, which will be the axis of your answer. So far you have Plano +/- _____ X 090. (You can't decide on the cylinder sign until you move to the next step.) For the next step, imagine that you are on a number line and have gone from zero to -2.25. How many steps from zero to -2.25? -2.25. That is your cylinder sign and power. The answer: Plano - 2.25 X 090. Of course, this could be transposed to - 2.25 + 2.25 X 180. Or you could have arrived at the plus cylinder answer by starting the process at the 180 meridian.

39. c) You can start in either meridian. Let's use -1.25. Now you know most of the answer: -1.25 +/- _____ X 135. How many steps to get from -1.25 to + 2.00? + 3.25. Finish it off: -1.25 + 3.25 X 135. However, this doesn't appear as an option in the answers listed. Instead, just transpose: + 2.00 - 3.25 X 045. (Transposition is a COA® level skill.)

40. d) The ocular media are the transparent structures of the eye through which light passes. Some references might not include the tear film. The term "the humors" refers to the aqueous humor and vitreous humor.

41. b) The cornea has more refractive power than even the lens. The average crystalline lens has 15 diopters of plus power. The cornea has 43.0.

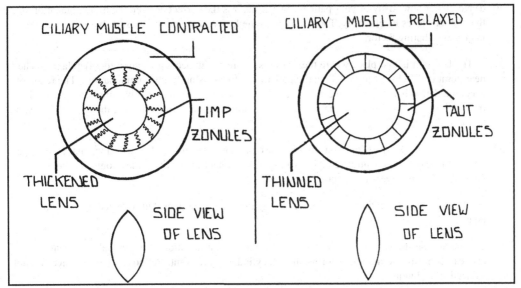

Figure 9-2. The lens and ciliary body in (a) accommodation and (b) relaxation. (Drawing by Holly Hess. Reprinted with permission from Ledford JK. *Exercises in Refractometry*. Thorofare, NJ: SLACK Incorporated; 1990.)

42. c) Incoming light is focused on the retina in the healthy eye. (Interpretation occurs in the occipital cortex of the brain.)

43. c) After the optic nerve, light impulses traverse the chiasm, optic tract, lateral geniculate body, and occipital cortex in that order. The brain stem, cerebral cortex, and cerebellum do not receive light impulses.

44. a) Figure 2-4 shows simple myopic astigmatism. Figure 2-5 depicts the corrected myopic portion with a minus sphere. But that pushes the emmetropic section back beyond the retina. So in Figure 2-6, a plus cylinder is used to pull that segment back onto the retina.

45. c) Figure 2-7 again shows simple myopic astigmatism. But this time, in Figure 2-8, it is corrected with a single minus cylinder. The cylinder moves only the myopic portion of the error, leaving the emmetropic section on the retina.

46. b) Figure 2-9 depicts mixed astigmatism. In Figure 2-10, the myopic portion is corrected with a minus sphere. This pushes the hyperopic segment even further from the retina. Figure 2-11 pulls the hyperopic rays forward onto the retina using plus cylinder, while leaving the already corrected portion undisturbed.

47. c) Figure 2-12 shows compound hyperopic astigmatism. Figure 2-13 shows a plus sphere pulling one meridian onto the retina. The other meridian is closer, but still not focused on the retina. So a plus cylinder is used, as in Figure 2-14, to pull that meridian the rest of the way.

48. c) The accommodative reflex (which is not a true physiologic reflex) operates for near vision, not distant.

49. c) When accommodation is relaxed, the ciliary muscle relaxes. This pulls the zonules tight, which stretches the lens out (thinning it). Distant objects become clear and the focusing power is decreased. See Figure 9-2.

50. d) No matter how many of your patients swear that *a* is the correct answer, the best explanation is that the lens loses its elasticity. There may be some laxity of the ciliary muscle, but this is not the major contributing factor.

51. a) The far point is that place where the vision is clearest with accommodation totally relaxed. The near point is the closest place where the patient can focus using full accommodation. The range of accommodation is the area between the near and far points. Accommodative amplitude is the dioptric value of the near point (ie, the amount of accommodation, in diopters, that the patient has available).

52. b) This was a tricky question. Your first impulse probably was to say "minus" since that is the type of lens that myopia is neutralized with. But in order to neutralize with minus, logically the eye must be plus. A myopic eye has too much plus power.

53. b) The light from the retinoscope is refracted by the cornea and lens, but reflected by the retina (specifically the pigment epithelium and choroid).

54. b) Rotating the streak of the streak retinoscope allows neutralization of individual meridians. You also can compare the meridians, or use minus cylinder if you want. Retinoscopy is an objective, not subjective, technique.

55. c) The streak retinoscope consists of a light source, power source, condensing lens, mirror, and focusing sleeve. There are no rotating lenses.

56. b) Moving the sleeve up and down changes the vergence of the light. One position has a plane mirror effect; the other has a concave effect. The position of the sleeve and its vergence varies from one brand of retinoscope to another.

57. c) When using the plane mirror effect, the light leaving the retinoscope is parallel. A concave mirror will focus the light in front of the instrument.

58. d) If a streak retinoscope is laid on its side while the bulb is hot, the filament can warp. This causes a C-shaped bend in the reflex.

59. a) Use of a working lens simulates infinity. This allows the technician to work at arm's length from the patient instead of 20 ft away.

60. b) Standard retinoscopy working distance is 66 cm (about 26 in) from the patient.

61. b) If your working distance is closer than 66 cm, you will need a stronger plus-power working lens.

62. d) The streak retinoscope allows for very accurate estimation of the cylinder axis.

63. d) The height of the streak is constant. Brightness, width, and speed of the moving reflex vary according to the patient's refractive error. A higher error will have a dull, narrow, and slow reflex.

64. d) The intercept is the part of the streak that falls on the patient's iris, or on the phoropter. It always travels in the direction in which you "sweep" (refers to moving the instrument back and forth) the scope. The light that shines from the pupil is called the reflex.

65. b) If the intercept and the reflex travel in the same direction, they are moving with each other. This is "with" motion. In "against" motion, the intercept moves in the opposite direction from the reflex. Neutrality just blinks on and off, while luminosity simply refers to the glow.

66. c) "With" motion is easier to see and interpret, regardless of what type of cylinder you use. Answers *a* and *b* refer to sphere sign, not cylinder.

67. d) Any situation can be converted to "with" motion. If you reduce the sphere enough (remove plus or add minus), "against" motion will convert to friendly "with".

68. a) In order to align the axis of the intercept with the angle of the reflex, turn the sleeve until there is an unbroken line (ie, the intercept and the reflex are aligned). Raising and lowering the sleeve changes the vergence of the scope's light.

69. b) A reflex that is approaching neutral will get brighter, wider, and faster.

70. c) At neutrality, the reflex will be its brightest, widest, and fastest. It will fill the whole pupil and appear to blink on and off.

71. d) Hold the scope with the right hand when using the right eye, and with the left hand when using the left eye. This makes it easier to turn the dials on the refractor. Statements *a* through *c* are true, although it takes some discipline to learn to work with both eyes open.

72. a) Rest the head of the retinoscope on your brow or against your glasses frame. This will help stabilize the instrument, keeping the peephole from wobbling around. It would be hard to manipulate the handle (raise, lower, or turn) if it were against your cheek. If you lean on the patient's chair, you are going to be too close. Resting it on the phoropter makes it impossible to work.

73. d) The undilated patient should look at a distant object in order to relax accommodation as much as possible. Options *a* through *c* are too close to the patient, and will stimulate accommodation. Looking at the retinoscopy light also will cause the pupil to constrict, making it harder to see the reflex.

74. c) A fully dilated patient can have some confusing reflexes. Concentrate on the central reflex, ignoring the periphery. There is no need to reduce the pupil size.

75. b) The streak should be moved ("swept") perpendicular to the intercept's direction. If the intercept is vertical, you move horizontally, and vice versa.

76. a) "Against" motion in all meridians indicates myopia. (Of course, it also could indicate compound myopic astigmatism, which wasn't given as an option.)

77. b) Mixed astigmatism has one focus in front of the retina (yielding "against" motion) and one behind the retina (giving "with" motion). Simple hyperopic astigmatism would have one neutral and one "with" meridian. Compound hyperopic astigmatism would have two "with" meridians. Compound myopic astigmatism would have two "against" meridians.

78. b) A high refractive error can masquerade as pseudo neutrality. Put in +5.00, +10.00, -5.00, and -10.00 spherical lenses and re-evaluate the reflex. The retinoscope is not generally used with the cross cylinder. Removing the working lens will only make a difference of 1.50 (or whatever the proper power is for your working distance), not enough to change the reflex much if evaluating a high refractive error.

79. a) One meridian is neutralized with plus, and the other meridian still has "with". Since you are using plus cylinder, and plus is used to neutralize "with", set your cylinder axis at 180 degrees and give plus cylinder until this meridian also is neutral.

80. c) The first "with" meridian is neutralized, and the other meridian still has "with" motion. Since you are using minus cylinder, you cannot neutralize "with" motion by using cylinder. If you neutralize the 135 meridian with sphere, this will convert the 045 meridian to "against". So neutralize 135 by adding more plus (or reducing minus). Then set your cylinder axis and retinoscope streak to 045. You will see "against". Give enough minus cylinder to convert this to "with", then reduce the amount of minus cylinder slowly until the meridian is neutralized.

81. c) If you are not using the built-in retinoscopy lens on the refractor, you must remember to subtract 1.50 sphere (or the appropriate amount for your personal working distance) from the measurement indicated on the refractor (ie, rotate the sphere wheel UP six "clicks" if your distance is 1.50).

82. c) None of these situations is ideal, but the patient with the IOL probably will be the easiest of the four to 'scope.

83. a) If the eye is fogged, how can the patient see to do the test? Fogging is used to reduce accommodation during refractometry, which helps prevent giving too much minus. It also can be used instead of occlusion.

84. c) To fog, add enough plus sphere to blur the vision. (There is no set amount, but I prefer +3.00.)

85. d) The astigmatic dial is useful in estimating the cylinder axis. You still must refine with the cross cylinder.

86. b) The astigmatic dial looks like a clock face.

87. c) If the lines on the dial appear equally black, add a little sphere (or move in a more plus direction) and ask again. (In minus cylinder, give -0.50.) Either way, you are moving the image off the retina enough to see if there is another meridian of focus.

88. a) For plus cylinder, set the cylinder axis parallel to (in line with) the darkest lines as the patient sees them.

89. d) In minus cylinder, set the cylinder axis perpendicular to (90 degrees away from) the darkest lines as the patient sees them.

90. a) After setting your axis, slowly give the patient cylinder power until the lines appear to be equally clear.

91. a) Use the cross cylinder to refine cylinder axis and power. (Spheres don't have an axis.)

92. a) If the spherical component of your measurement is too far off, your cylinder won't be correct. You'll be trying to correct things with cylinder that would be corrected better with sphere.

93. d) Always measure the cylinder axis first. (This is one of the few exceptions to my warning about the word *always*.) If the axis isn't refined first, you can't get the accurate power. Doing this in the wrong order used to be grounds for failing the refractometry section of the practical; it remains to be seen how the "virtual practical" will see things.

94. a) If you are using minus cylinder and are refining axis, follow the red dot. (There are no blue dots.)

95. c) When refining power, the red dot means subtract (same as "giving minus") and the white dot means add (same as "giving plus"), regardless of whether you are working in plus or minus cylinder. If you are at cylinder power +0.50 and the patient likes the white dot choice better, you are going to move to +1.00 cylinder power. (In reality, you could alternately choose to go to +0.75, adding just +0.25, but that was not offered as an answer in this question.)

96. c) See above. The white dot means give plus, so you should move from -1.00 to -0.50.

97. c) The cross cylinder actually straddles a setting, so on one choice the patient sees the setting with a little "plus", and on the other choice with a little "minus". When straddling the correct reading, each choice is equidistant from that setting and the choices will look about the same.

98. a) Green rays are refracted more than red rays, so red hits the retina first. Adding minus moves the red rays behind the retina, and pulls the green forward onto the retina. There is a difference of 0.50 - 0.75 diopters between the red and green wavelengths. Colors do not appear as other colors. Normal color vision is not required (see question 103). *Note*: The duochrome test may also be called the bichrome test.

99. c) The duochrome test is used to prevent giving the patient too much minus sphere. It is not a color vision test, nor is it used to refine cylinder. (The only time you have to worry about giving too much *plus* is when measuring the reading add.)

100. c) The red filter is not used in the duochrome test. Fogging the eye with +0.50 makes the letters in the red darker, so you can move toward the green by -0.25 steps.

101. d) If the letters in the red are sharper and more distinct, remove 0.25 diopters of sphere (ie, reduce plus or increase minus). Go in small steps so you don't miss the end point and over minus.

102. c) The end point is when the letters on both sides are equally clear.

103. d) Even a red-green color blind patient who cannot distinguish between vivid hues can be tested using the duochrome if you refer to the left and right halves of the screen instead of the colors. No special lenses or tricks need to be used.

104. b) If the patient accommodates, he has added plus power to the eye. This is neutralized with minus sphere (or the removal of plus sphere) during the measurement. If prescribed by the practitioner, this spectacle lens won't have enough plus, and the eye will have to strain when wearing it. (And even *more* accommodation will be required for clear vision.)

105. b) Methods to control or reduce accommodation include the duochrome test, fogging, and topical cycloplegics. Bringing the distant chart closer will stimulate accommodation.

106. c) See question 104.

107. b) It is a common misconception that if the patient is known to be myopic, you need not worry about accommodation. This isn't true. You might easily refract a young myope who only needs -2.00 sphere as a -4.00 or more.

108. d) As a general rule, the ideal situation for distance is for accommodation to be relaxed and vision to be as clear as possible.

109. a) The history will tell you much that can affect the measurement: the presence of any systemic or ocular disease that may affect vision, any medications that can affect vision, past vision history, past problems with glasses, visual symptoms, etc. The option of doing a slit lamp exam prior to refractometry is preferable, but not as necessary as knowing the patient's history.

110. d) As a general rule, taking allergy shots does not affect the measurement. Items *a*, *b*, and *c* can change the measurement.

111. a) Refractometry should be done prior to tonometry or any other procedure that applanates the cornea (A-scan, B-scan, pachymetry, cell count, etc.). With any of these tests there is the possibility of some corneal abrasion and/or edema, which can affect the patient's vision and thus the measurement. The pupil test might dazzle the patient for a minute, but you can proceed once he recovers. Dilation should be done after distance and near testing, but will not "contaminate" the distance measurement.

112. c) The slit lamp exam will indicate the clarity of the tear film, cornea, aqueous, lens, and vitreous (collectively called the *optical media*), giving you an idea of the prognosis of the measurement. Unless the patient has marked keratoconus, astigmatism will not be seen with the slit lamp. Applanation tonometry was ruled out in the last question. The necessity for a measurement is normally determined by factors other than the slit lamp exam.

113. c) Refractometry is the measurement of a patient's refractive error (by objective and/or subjective means), and usually is recorded in the patient's chart. Refraction includes the clinical judgment necessary to arrive at the prescription based on the refractometric measurement. Ophthalmic medical personnel are allowed to perform refractometry. Refractions are done only by those licensed to practice medicine.

114. a) Patient education is one of the keys to successful measurements. An auto-refractor reading might be nice, but is not necessary. Obviously not everyone can read 20/20 (or they wouldn't need us). If the tear film is cloudy, teardrops may be needed, but they are not needed on every patient.

115. d) A patient with head tremors will be easier to work with using the trial frame. It would be difficult to keep such a patient aligned with the refractor. A patient with facial deformities may not be able to wear or tolerate a trial frame. Retinoscopy is more conveniently done using the refractor.

116. Labeling:

PD adjusting knob	j
Cylinder power	a
Cylinder power dial	o
Prism	m
PD scale	g
Sphere dial	d
Aperture convergence level	f
Cross cylinder	l
Sphere power	c
3 diopter sphere dial	k
Level	i
Aperture	b
Cylinder axis dial	n
Aperture knob	e
Leveling screw	h

117. c) Always set the PD, vertex distance, and level before measuring. The apertures are converged to test the reading (near) vision, not the distance.

118. b) The measurement starts by working with spheres. You want to correct as much of the refractive error with spheres (instead of sometimes poorly tolerated cylinder) as possible.

119. b) Always offer more plus first, whether you are going from +2.00 to +2.50, or from -6.25 to -5.75. More minus always will look better to an eye that is accommodating. Sphere has no axis.

120. d) If sphere alone does not correct a patient to 20/20, it is not time to stop! Start looking for astigmatism. If -2.00 and -2.50 sphere did not improve, it is a waste of time to try -1.75 and -2.25. The duochrome test is performed once best visual acuity has been obtained using spheres and, if necessary, cylinder.

121. a) For every 0.50 diopter of minus cylinder, you should now add 0.25 diopters of sphere. This is to maintain equivalence. (In plus cylinder, for every 0.50 diopters of cylinder, you should *subtract* 0.25 diopters of sphere.)

122. c) Remember that a minus lens minifies. (You also could say that, compared to a +6.00, a +2.00 minifies.) The patient's impression that the letters have gotten smaller is an indication of too much minus. Therefore, you return to the previous setting of -2.00 + 1.25 X 065 as your end point.

123. c) Any time a healthy-looking eye does not refract to 20/20, do a pinhole vision. If the pinhole improves the vision, you should be able to improve it with the correct lenses. If the pinhole does not improve the vision, your refractometric measurement is probably the best you can do, and the doctor will look for pathology.

124. d) Cylinder power in most refractors goes up to 6.00 diopters, but there is an auxiliary cylinder lens that you can snap into the aperture to add more. The cross cylinder is not dependent on a certain amount of astigmatism.

125. c) Both eyes are open during balancing. (Standing on one foot?!? I thought it was time for a little levity; optics can get pretty heavy!)

126. b) The goal in balancing is to make sure that the eyes are accommodating equally. (Ideally, of course, this means that neither eye is accommodating at all.)

127. c) The refractometrist should measure the add at 14 inches, and make a note for the practitioner as to the distance preferred by the patient.

128. a) In general, be cautious with giving plus and also to leave half of the patient's accommodation in reserve. If you give the maximum plus that the patient will tolerate, you totally eliminate natural accommodation at near. The age chart may be a guide, but each patient should be measured. Some patients will need more than +3.00. The word "never" should have indicated that this choice was not correct.

129. c) Use larger steps for low vision patients to provide more contrast between the compared lenses. No need to speak louder; they can hear. Go more slowly, rather than quickly. Small steps are harder for them to see and judge.

130. c) Of the listed procedures, a nasolacrimal probing is least likely to produce a change in refractometry. Pterygium removal may alter the cornea. Heavy lids may press on the globe, as may a chalazion.

131. a) A patient with a progressive cataract usually begins to take more minus (or less plus).

132. c) Elevated blood sugar causes a *myopic* shift. Fluid leaves the lens as the body attempts to neutralize the sugar in the blood. This dehydration causes an increase in the lens's curve, resulting in a myopic shift. The items in *a*, *b*, and *d* can cause a hyperopic shift.

133. a) See question 132.

134. b) Keratoconus causes shifts in astigmatism as it progresses. Astigmatism itself, in the absence of keratoconus or physical alteration of the cornea, generally remains stable. Contact lens overwear causes more pain than refractive change. Glaucoma does not generally cause a change in the refractometric measurement.

135. c) The effective diameter (ED) of a lens is measured diagonally (one corner to the other) across the eyewire opening of the frame. Add 2 mm to this measurement to determine the size of lens blank needed for the frame. (If the lens is decentered, you must add this in as well.)

136. b) The closer one gets to the cornea (or retina, for that matter), the higher the lens power must be. This occurs because the focal length has been shortened. See questions 137 to 141.

137. a) Vertex distance is the distance from the back of the corrective lens to the front of the cornea.

138. c) Vertex distance is more crucial in high-powered lenses. The weaker the lens, the more "play" there is in the allowable vertex distance.

139. c) If the patient's refractive error is 4.00 diopters (plus or minus) or more, you should measure vertex distance and record this in the chart for the prescriber. Some references may say 3.00 diopters or more.

140. b) A distometer is used to measure vertex distance. A vertexometer is a type of lensometer, used to measure the refractive power of a lens. Ophthalmometer is another name for keratometer.

141. a) If you want to convert a lens power for a given vertex distance (or vice versa), you must use a conversion scale. Some are tables and others are rotary-type charts.

142. a) The lens may not read as being exactly what the doctor ordered if the optician had to adjust for vertex distance. Diplopia and induced prism are a function of optical center alignment. Vision should be just as good regardless.

143. a) Because prism displaces the apparent location of an object, it is used in ophthalmic lenses to redirect the line of sight. Prisms cannot function in *b*, *c*, or *d*. (They are used to *treat* strabismus, but cannot *cure* it.)

144. c) There is no such thing as a power compensation prism.

145. b) A person can overcome a horizontal imbalance of some magnitude, but only can overcome a vertical imbalance of less than 1.00 prism diopter. The patient in answer *c* probably won't have any problem, first, because both eyes are myopic, and second, because 1.00 diopter isn't that great a difference. Intermittent esotropia is straight much of the time; the patient has some ability to overcome it.

146. a) Press-on prisms are ideal for temporary use, as in a recovering nerve palsy. The other situations listed in *b*, *c*, and *d* are long-term.

147. b) If the optical centers are displaced nasally, they are decentered inward.

148. a) A minus lens is like two prisms placed apex to apex. If the optical center of the left lens is moved to the left, this means that the eye is looking through the lens to the right of the optical center through the prism, which is base in.

149. c) A plus lens is like two prisms placed base to base. The right eye is looking under the "line" where the bases meet, so it gets the effect of base up. The left eye is looking over the "line" where the bases meet, so it gets the effect of base down.

150. a) It is common to split higher degrees of prism between the two eyes. Horizontal prism diopters placed in the same direction are additive.

151. d) Vertical prism is additive if placed in *opposite* directions. Situation *c* would move the eyes farther apart.

152. d) Prentice's rule says that displacement (in cm) X lens power (in diopters) = power of induced prism.

153. a) The induced prismatic effect of a lens in prism diopters equals the power of the lens (in diopters) multiplied by the displacement of the optical centers (in cm). Thus, 4.25 x 0.50 = 2.125. As to base placement, see question 149.

154. c) Using the above formula, 3.0 = 6.50 x ?. Divide both sides by 6.5, and you get 0.46 cm. But all the answers were in mm. There are 10 mm in 1 cm, so 0.46 cm = 4.6 mm. Moving the center down has the effect of moving the optical axis up. In a minus lens, this produces base up prism.

155. a) First, plus lenses that are decentered *in* will induce base in prism. Since both lenses are base in, their power is additive. Next, figure the induced prism in each lens. OD: prism = 2.75 x .275 = 0.75 induced prism diopters. OS: prism = 2.00 x .125 = 0.25 induced prism diopters. Add the induced prism OD and OS: 0.75 + 0.25 = 1.00 prism diopters base in.

156. d) The weaker the lens, the less induced prism there is if it is decentered (regardless of direction). For example, 0.50 cm decentration will induce 6 prism diopters in the +12.00 lens, 3 diopters in the -6.00 lens, 2 diopters in the +4.00 lens, and 1 diopter in the -2.00 lens.

157. c) Anisometropia (a difference of over 1.00 diopter between eyes) can induce prism and unwanted diplopia for near vision.

158. a) A slab-off (bicentric) lens is an aid for near vision, nothing else.

159. d) The patient should be educated in *a* through *c* before given the prescription. The slab-off should not affect the visual acuity for better or worse, but will make the patient more comfortable and get rid of the double vision.

160. b) To make the slab-off, a portion of the near vision segment is ground away.

161. c) The slab-off process moves the optical center of the reading segment closer to that of the upper distant segment.

162. b) The first step in helping patients adapt to anything is educating them so they have realistic expectations. Let them know about the problems inherent with aphakic correction ahead of time.

163. b) Magnification is a characteristic of plus lenses. (Minification and "with" motion are characteristics of *minus,* or concave, lenses.) When objects appear to be larger than they actually are, they also appear to be closer. This throws off depth perception.

164. a) A lenticular lens has an optical portion ground onto a carrier.

165. c) As its name implies, the full-field lens offers a larger field of view.

166. d) A lenticular lens looks sort of like a fried egg (not very appealing on one's face).

167. b) PD and vertex distance are critical in every high-powered lens, regardless of type.

168. c) The spectacle-ring scotoma is a problem in high plus lenses regardless of material.

169. d) The higher the power of the lens, the more critical it is to provide an accurate PD and vertex distance. Without the PD, you may have induced prism. Without the correct vertex distance, the lens power may not be adequate.

170. a) The combination of the lenticular form with aspheric surfaces eliminates most of the problems inherent with high plus lenses.

171. a) The two main types of low vision aids are optical and nonoptical. Items in answer *b* are nonoptical aids, and items in answers *c* and *d* are optical aids.

172. a) Examples of optical aids include magnifiers, telescopes, high-powered bifocals, and stand magnifiers. Large print, yellow filters, Braille, high-intensity lamps, CCTV, and books on tape are nonoptical. Answer *a* was the only option that offered *only* optical aids.

173. b) Nonoptical aids include those mentioned above, plus writing and reading guides. Answer *b* is the only list of nonoptical aids without any optical aids thrown in.

174. b) Minifying the distant scene for a visual field impaired person shrinks the view to within his available field.

175. c) Any type of magnifying system enlarges the image that falls on the retina.

176. b) A working distance of 40 cm (16 inches) is the basis for the manufacturing of low vision magnifiers. Since the 40 cm is the current standard, it will be used in the remainder of this text. *Note:* Some manufacturers base their lens power on a standard of 25 cm (10 inches) rather than 40. This is also referred to as "X". Yes, it is confusing. And yes, it can lead to incorrect powers when ordering low vision aids. You should read the dioptric power of any magnifier you order to be sure it is what the patient needs.

177. c) To find the dioptric power of a magnifier, multiply the "X" power by 2.5. 10 x 2.5 = 25 diopters.

178. c) To find the magnifying power of the lens, first convert that working distance to dioptric power. Figure your focal length: a 5 cm working distance requires a 20 diopter lens (100/5 = 20). To ascertain the "X" notation, divide the dioptric power by 2.5 (20/2.5 = 8).

179. a) This is a simple focal length question. 100 cm/30 D = 3.33 cm.

180. a) A telescope that has been modified for near work allows the user to have a greater working distance than with magnifiers.

181. b) A person with a hand tremor would have trouble holding a hand magnifier still. The other three options don't require the user to hold anything.

182. d) CCTV allows a wide range of magnification capabilities combined with being able to save the reading material on disk.

183. b) Illumination in the office situation is set up to be ideal. Lighting at home is often less than ideal. Patients should be instructed as to the proper lighting to use with every visual aid sent home.

Chapter 3. Basic Ocular Motility

1. b) Adduction means the eye is turning in toward the nose. Abduction is turning out, or away. (Remember, if someone is abducted, they are taken away.)

2. d) Depression refers to turning down.

3. a) The only muscles that have a primary action and no other are the MR and LR, which adduct and abduct respectively. (The other four muscles have secondary and tertiary actions as well as a primary action.)

4. c) The IO and SR act to elevate the eye, the IO in adduction and the SR in abduction.

5. b) The obliques abduct as a tertiary action. (Memory hint: oBliques aBduct.)

6. d) The primary action of the oblique muscles is torsional. The SO intorts and the IO extorts.

7. a) The eye's depressors are the IR and SO. The IR depresses in abduction and the SO depresses in adduction.

8. a) The SR and IR (ie, both vertical rectus muscles) have the tertiary action of adduction.

9. a) Yoked muscles are muscles in each eye that accomplish the same version movement. In the examples given, the RLR and LMR both accomplish right gaze. The RLR and RMR are in the same eye, which doesn't fulfill the definition. The combinations of RLR and LLR, and RIR and LIR accomplish vergences, not versions.

10. d) A synergist is a muscle in the same eye that assists another muscle in accomplishing a particular action. The muscles that help the MR in horizontal movement are the SR (in upgaze) and IR (in downgaze).

11. b) An antagonist is a muscle in the same eye that works against a particular action. The muscles that work against depression by the IR are the SR and IO, both of which are elevators.

12. c) Unless it is intermittent, a tropia is there all the time. If you can look at the patient and see that one eye is turned, it is a tropia. "Lazy eye" is the layman's term for amblyopia. A phoria is evident only when you cover one eye or otherwise disrupt fusion.

13. b) A phoria is evident only when you disrupt fusion. *Note*: Some phorias "break down" when the patient is tired. This is actually an intermittent deviation.

14. d) A phoria usually is controlled unless fusion is disrupted. When the disruption is removed, the eyes will fuse again. An intermittent tropia comes and goes; sometimes the patient is fusing and sometimes he's not. When he's not fusing, the deviation appears.

15. c) An adult with a crossed eye either has learned to suppress the image from the eye that is not fixating or he has double vision (if he has not learned or is unable to suppress). It is not a given that amblyopia or anisometropia exist, although they might. Fusion and stereopsis can occur only when both eyes are working together, looking at the same object.

16. Labeling on Figure 3-1:
    Esotropia   b
    Exotropia   d
    Hypertropia   c
    Hypotropia   e
    Orthophoria   a

17. b) Reading would *encourage* fusion (at least until fatigue sets in), as it causes convergence.

18. a) If convergence is insufficient, the patient is not able to pull the eyes inward for near viewing. Thus, the deviation is greater at near than at a distance. *Note*: Convergence insufficiency also can occur in orthophoria.

19. b) A convergence excess means that the eyes overconverge for near viewing. Thus, an esotropia would be worse at near in this situation.

20. a) In an A pattern, the eyes are more converged in upgaze and more diverged in downgaze. A V pattern is more diverged in upgaze and more converged in downgaze. They *can* be measured with prisms.

21. c) The secondary and tertiary actions of the IO are elevation and abduction. Because the IO has its action in upgaze, an overaction would likely increase abduction, hence the V pattern.

22. b) In order of *decreasing* occurrence: V pattern ET, V pattern XT, A pattern ET, and A pattern XT.

23. d) Congenital anisometropia (unequal refractive errors) leads to amblyopia. The eye that requires the least amount of accommodation for the best vision is the eye that will be used. There is a general tendency for an amblyopic eye to drift out (ie, be exotropic), rather than in. (Obviously, this is not always the case, but it is the most common.)

24. d) In an orbital blow-out fracture, the muscles become entrapped in the lower orbit, restricting vertical movement. The situation in answers *a* or *c* may lead to an exodeviation (an unused eye tends to drift outward). Down's syndrome is associated with esotropia, also a horizontal deviation.

25. a) Conventionally, vertical deviations are described as a hypertropia of the higher eye. Thus, if the patient was fixating with the right eye and the left eye was deviated downward, the right eye is higher. So this situation would be designated as an RHT.

26. a) Duane's syndrome causes a horizontal deviation.

27. a) In a vertical deviation one eye is higher than the other, thus the doubled images are one above the other or possibly diagonal to each other. A horizontal deviation causes doubled images that are beside each other.

28. d) The prefix "pseudo" means false. Thus, pseudostrabismus is false strabismus; the eyes falsely appear to be crossed although they are straight.

29. c) Because infants have a flat nasal bridge and (sometimes) epicanthal folds, they are implicated more often in pseudostrabismus (an optical illusion of esotropia) than any other group. There is no indication whether boys or girls are most often affected.

30. a) See question 29.

31. d) An incomitant (or noncomitant) deviation varies according to the patient's field of gaze. A comitant deviation is the same in all fields of gaze.

32. b) An adult or child with a *new* nerve palsy notices double vision. (A child with a congenital nerve palsy learns to suppress one image and does not see double.)

33. b) If the muscle is not getting a full nerve supply, it will not be able to react properly (if at all). It thus will be underactive. This might manifest itself as an overaction of the muscle's antagonist.

34. c) Ductions are movements of one eye. If you have determined that a phoria exists and you suspect it to be a nerve palsy, test the fields of gaze of one eye at a time while covering the nontested eye. If the deviation is *not* paralytic, each eye will have full range of motion. In a paralytic deviation, the affected eye will not have full range of motion.

35. b) If the patient has paralytic strabismus and you measure the deviation, the deviation will be larger when the patient is fixating with the affected eye. This is called the secondary deviation. (The measurement derived while fixing with the unaffected eye is the primary deviation.)

36. c) See question 35.

37. b) See question 35.

38. a) If there is a palsy of the LR, whose only action is abduction, then the gaze most affected by the condition will be abduction.

39. c) If the SO is palsied, the direction of gaze that will be most affected is down and in (which is also the field of gaze in which you test SO action).

40. a) The SO is the only EOM enervated by the fourth cranial nerve. Because of the nerve's positioning, a bilateral SO palsy is commonly associated with head trauma.

41. b) The B3ST is used to isolate the cyclovertical muscle (IR, SR, IO, SO) that is causing a paralytic strabismus. (If the paralysis occurs in the LR or MR it is obvious because these two muscles have only one action each.)

42. c) The B3ST is most accurate on new cases of paralytic strabismus because the deviations in various fields of gaze are more sharply defined. After a period of time, these boundaries begin to blur as there is a "spread of comitance," or a tendency for the deviations to become more alike in various fields of gaze.

43. b) Each step of the B3ST rules out certain muscles as the paralyzed muscle. The first step of the B3ST consists of determining which eye is higher (hypertropic) in primary gaze. An RHT implicates RIR/RSO and LIO/LSR. An LHT implicates RSR/RIO and LSO/LIR.

44. d) The second step of the B3ST is to determine if the hypertropia is worse in left or right gaze. Worse in right gaze implicates RSR/RIR and LIO/LSO. Worse in left gaze implicates RIO/RSO and LSR/LIR.

45. b) Step 3 of the B3ST consists of determining if the hypertropia is worse when the head is *tilted* (not turned) to the left or the right. Worse in right head tilt implicates RSR/RSO and LIO/LIR. Worse in left tilt implicates RIR/RIO and LSO/LSR.

46. a) Step 1: RHT implicates RIR/RSO and LIO/LSR. Step 2: Worse in right gaze implicates RSR/RIR and LIO/LSO. Step 3: Worse in left tilt implicates RIO/RSO and LSR/LIR. The muscle with three "hits" is the RIR.

47. b) The common lay-term for amblyopia is lazy eye. But if a parent tells you that a child has a lazy eye, have the parent define it for you. She may be referring to an eye that drifts in or out (strabismus) or to a drooping eyelid (ptosis). "Walleyed" refers to an exodeviation, and "cross-eyed" refers to an esodeviation or to strabismus in general.

48. d) Amblyopia occurs in an eye that never learns how to see. Even after any organic problem is resolved, corrective lenses still will not improve vision. Answer *a* is the definition of abnormal retinal correspondence.

49. b) In situation b, the brain will only accommodate enough to focus the least hyperopic eye, leaving the +4.00 eye in a constant blur and in danger of becoming amblyopic. The 3-year-old in answer *a* is likely to use the -3.00 eye for near (as it requires no accommodation) and the +0.50 eye for distant visual activities. Although amblyopia *could* occur in such a scenario, it is much more likely in hyperopic anisometropia. Amblyopia develops by age 12, not after. A single mm of ptosis is not enough to drop the lid over the pupil. (If the lid covers the pupil, then amblyopia of disuse could develop.)

50. b) If the child alternates, it means he is using one eye as much as the other. The conclusion is that the vision must be about equal in either eye. The child would not choose to use an amblyopic eye.

51. a) If the eyes are best corrected and there is a difference of two or more acuity lines in the vision of the eyes, the diagnosis is amblyopia. An amblyopic patient will fail the stereo test, but so will other patients with other eye problems.

52. c) An amblyopic eye can identify figures more easily if they are isolated than if they are presented in a group. This is called the *crowding phenomenon*. An accurate vision on an amblyopic eye can be obtained only by using a row of age-appropriate figures.

53. b) Rating an infant's vision as central, steady, and maintained is not useful in diagnosing amblyopia. Even an eye with poor vision can maintain steady central looking. In the 25 diopter prism test, base in, the prism is held over one eye then the other. A child with equal vision in each eye will use the eye without the prism to fixate regardless of which eye is looking through the prism. While the PL and VEP do not give an actual acuity level, they *can* identify a difference in acuity between the two eyes, which strongly indicates amblyopia.

54. c) The occluder is used in strabismus cover tests to disrupt fusion, ie, to prevent the eyes from being locked onto the same target. Fusion will hold a phoria and often an intermittent deviation in check, so fusion must be disrupted in order to determine if these deviations exist.

55. c) The cover tests are objective; they are based on the observations of the examiner rather than on the responses of the subject. Thus, they can be performed on an infant or any other patient who cannot or will not give a verbal response.

56. d) There is no point in doing cover tests on a monocular patient because there is no vision in the second eye with which to fuse. The patient must always fixate with the single, seeing eye.

57. a) The cover/uncover test differentiates between a phoria and a tropia.

58. a) The cover/uncover test also indicates the direction of any deviation (ie, eso, exo, or vertical).

59. c) The eyes must have drifted *out* under the cover if they make *inward* movements when uncovered, so an exodeviation is present. You were not given enough information to differentiate between a phoria and tropia. For that, you need to know what the uncovered eye is doing, as well.

60. d) An *outward* motion upon uncovering indicates that the eye has drifted *in*, denoting an esodeviation. In this case, regardless of which eye is covered, the covered eye drifts in. When the eye is uncovered, it does not move to take up fixation (indicating a tropia). This further indicates that the patient is willing to use either eye to fix, revealing an alternating esotropia.

61. c) In a phoria, the eye under the cover drifts. The eye that is not covered is fixating. When you remove the cover, the resulting diplopia causes the deviated eye to move in order to pick up fixation. The eye that was not covered is fixating already, so it does not need to move. Be sure to read the questions carefully; the answer would have been different if this had been a cross cover test.

62. d) The alternate (or cross) cover test will reveal horizontal and vertical deviations, but does not differentiate between a phoria and a tropia.

63. b) When performing the alternate (cross) cover test, move the cover rapidly from one eye to the other, but every half-second is too fast. The important thing is to prevent the patient from seeing with both eyes at once, thus regaining fusion.

64. b) If no motion is seen during the alternate (cross) cover test, it is logical to assume that the patient is orthophoric. You cannot, however, assume that amblyopia does or does not exist, that the patient has stereopsis, or that vision is equal in both eyes.

65. d) The only thing you know at this point is that there is some type of exodeviation. (For the eye to move inward when it is uncovered, it must have drifted outward under the cover.) Once you have found movement on the alternate (cross) cover test, use the cover/uncover test to determine if it is a tropia or a phoria.

66. c) The alternate cover test combined with prisms to measure the size of a deviation (phoria or tropia) becomes a prism and cover test. The deviation can be measured in a patient with fusion because the test itself disrupts fusion. The corneal reflex and polarized glasses are not used in the prism and cover test.

67. b) It doesn't matter over which eye the prism is held. Statements *a, c,* and *d* are true.

68. a) The prism's apex should point in the same direction as the deviation. You've probably been taught that the base goes in the opposite direction as the deviation. That's just a different way to say the same thing. (Think of the prism as an arrow in order to help you remember which way to use the prism.) For measuring, it is not necessary (or practical) to split the prism amount between the two eyes. The prism may be placed over either eye.

69. b) The end point is reached when you have added prism sufficient enough so that neither eye moves when you cross cover. (Except for paralytic strabismus, the eyes move an equal amount anyway.) Answers *c* and *d* are wrong because the prism and cover test is objective, not subjective.

70. d) The patient has an RHT; the right eye is higher, so the prism apex ("arrow") should point up. This puts the base *down.* You could put the prism in front of the left eye, too, but the left is the lower eye so the apex would point down (ie, base up). This was not offered as an answer.

71. d) The patient has a 15 diopter ET. The prisms are base out, with the apexes "pointing" to the nasal. This indicates that you are dealing with an esodeviation. The power of the prisms is additive, hence 15 diopters.

72. d) This question is tough; I had to draw it out to make sure I wrote it correctly. First, vertical is being dealt with, so one eye has to be up and the other has to be down. But both prisms are in the same position. In a vertical deviation, this means they are *not* additive because one negates the other (at least as much as it is able to, power-wise). Remaining are 10 diopters of prism power that actually are working (15-5=10). Since the prism over the right eye is stronger, that is the prism that remains effective. A 10 diopter prism base up over the right eye remains. The apex is pointing down, indicating that the right eye is hypotropic, meaning that the left eye is hypertropic. Since vertical deviations are usually labeled by indicating the higher eye, this is a 10 diopter LHT. (Feel free to draw little pictures on your scratch paper during the exam.)

73. c) The Hirschberg and Krimsky tests both involve the location of a light reflex on the patient's cornea or sclera. While the patient fixates on your nose or another object, the penlight is used to create the reflex. The tests do not involve pupillary reaction or evaluate muscle action.

74. b) In an orthophoric patient the reflexes are normally a bit nasal in each eye, as shown in the top pair of eyes in Figure 3-1 (question 16). There are exceptions, but the main point is that the reflex should fall in the same place on each eye in orthophoria.

75. c) The reflex is displaced in OS. An inward reflex indicates an eye that deviates outward, so this is an LXT. The general rule for the Hirschberg is that 1 mm of displacement equals 15 prism diopters. A light reflex at the pupillary margin of a 4 mm pupil has been displaced about 2 mm, indicating a 30 prism diopter (Δ) turn. A light reflex halfway across the iris indicates 60 Δ, and at the outer edge of the limbus (as in this case), it would be 90 Δ.

76. b) The reflex is displaced out, OD, indicating an RET. The reflex falls halfway across the iris, giving an estimated 60 Δ deviation.

77. a) The reflex is displaced in, OS, indicating an LXT. The reflex is at pupil's edge, so the estimate is 30 Δ.

78. d) Cooperative binocular patients can have their deviations measured more precisely than a Hirschberg test. For bedside evaluation (no prisms available), the Hirschberg is great. On an infant that doesn't like bright lights, a quick Hirschberg estimate is all you may get. A patient with a blind eye cannot fixate to do cover tests, and in most cases a precise measurement is not required (unless cosmetic straightening is to be done).

79. b) The Krimsky measurement involves moving the Hirschberg reflexes by means of prisms. No occluder, special glasses, or Maddox rod are needed.

80. d) In the Krimsky test, prisms are used to move the displaced reflex to a position that is relative to the reflex on the fixating eye. No cover testing is used, nor is fixation of both eyes required. The Krimsky will likely give a more accurate measurement than the Hirschberg estimation, so the numbers may not match exactly.

81. Matching:
    A. Up and right   c
    B. Straight ahead   a
    C. Up   b
    D. Down and left   c
    E. Up and left   c
    F. Right   b
    G. Down and right   c
    H. Left   b
    I. Down   b

82. c) Straight ahead (primary gaze), straight up, and straight down are not cardinal positions of gaze. In any of these positions, the action of one muscle can be masked by the action of another, so these positions are not considered diagnostic.

83. b) When testing versions (range of motion), it is important that the patient keep his head still. If the patient moves the head to follow the target, you are not able to test the full motion of the eyes, but rather the range of motion of the neck! The test is done in room light so you can see the eyes as they move. An occluder is not used when testing versions. If the eyes remained in primary position, they would not move at all.

84. b) Looking down and right (from the *patient's* perspective) requires the RIR and LSO. Straight ahead (primary gaze) is not diagnostic. RSR and LIO are up and right. RSO and LIR are down and left. See Figure 9-3 on the next page.

Figure 9-3. Pairs of yoke muscles responsible for moving eyes into various positions of gaze. Reprinted from Hansen V. *A Systematic Approach to Strabismus*. Thorofare, NJ: SLACK Incorporated; 1998.

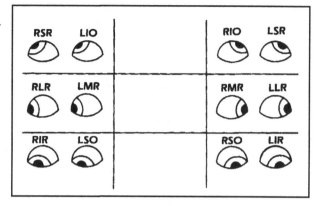

85. b) In down and left gaze, the RSO and LIR are being utilized. RIR and LSO would be down and right. RSR and LIO are up and right. RIO and LSR are up and left.

86. b) The RLR has its primary action in right gaze. Left gaze would be the RMR. Down and right would be RIR, and up and left would be RIO.

87. d) To check the action of the LIO, have the patient look up and right. Left gaze would check the LLR. Down and right would be the LSO, and up and left would be the LSR.

88. c) The Maddox rod test can be used to measure both phorias (because it disrupts fusion) and tropias. It is used to evaluate horizontal and vertical deviations.

89. c) The Maddox rod test requires a cooperative, honest patient who does not suppress. (A patient who suppresses would not see the red line, nor would a monocular patient, when the rod was placed over the blind eye.)

90. b) The Maddox rod test can be performed in all positions of gaze at distance and at near. It is a subjective measurement, not objective, because it depends on the response of the subject.

91. c) The red line appears perpendicular to the direction of the rods. If the rods are vertical, the line is horizontal.

92. a) A horizontal line is used to measure a vertical deviation, because the line can then be moved up and down. A vertical line is used to measure a horizontal deviation, because the line can then be moved left and right.

93. a) The Maddox rod is placed over the nonfixating eye and the prism is placed over the rod. An occluder is not used, and individual prisms are easier to hold.

94. b) The eye behind the Maddox rod sees a red line, while the other eye sees the light source. Orthophoria is reached when the red line goes through the light.

95. d) If the rod is placed so that the ridges are vertical, then the line is running horizontally, which checks for a vertical deviation, not a horizontal deviation such as an ET.

96. b) The ridges are horizontal, creating a vertical line for checking horizontal deviations. You have placed the rod in front of the left eye, and the line is to the right. This indicates a left exotropia. If the line were to the left, a left esotropia would be indicated.

97. a) The above situation, where the image is on the side opposite to the eye viewing through the Maddox rod, is referred to as *crossed diplopia*. If the line were on the left, there would be *uncrossed diplopia*. Vertical deviation is not being tested in this case. The Maddox rod does not work in a patient with suppression.

98. d) Since the patient has an exodeviation, the prism would be placed base in (or apex "arrow" pointing out, in the direction of the deviation).

99. b) Properly performed, the W4D can indicate all items in answers *a*, *c*, and *d*. Fusional amplitudes are the patient's vergence ability.

100. c) If the patient can distinguish between the two colors, the W4D can be performed. Additionally, he must be able to count objects ("How many dots do you see?") However, being able to count is not enough; the patient must be able to reliably count objects. Believe it or not, normal color vision is not required because even the red/green color deficient patient can distinguish between the colors. It is the examiner's job to interpret the patient's responses. Even knowing left from right isn't needed if you tap the patient's right hand and say, "Are the red lights on this side," then tap the left hand and say, "or on this side?" Literacy is not required, either.

101. b) The standard test screen or flashlight has two green, one red, and one white light.

102. a) By convention, the flashlight is held with the white light at the bottom. This puts the red light on the top, and a green light on either side.

103. b) Again, by convention, the glasses are placed on the patient with the red lens over the right eye. (I remember this by the R's: Right, Red.) The patient with fusion will report seeing four lights.

104. c) A patient who fuses may report any of the listed combinations *except* for seeing one red light on the bottom and three green lights (on top, left, and right). Additionally, sometimes the bottom light might be seen as yellowish, a sort of blended red and green.

105. d) The eye looking through the red lens (usually OD) will see the red light as red, and the white light as red. The two green lights are not seen. The eye looking through the green lens (usually OS) will see the two green lights as green, and the white light as green. The single red light is not visible. Thus, the patient in the example is suppressing with the left eye.

106. a) Once the patient reports seeing five lights, determine if there is alternate suppression present before going any further. If there is, then the patient will alternately see two reds then three greens. If there is not, then diplopia exists, and you should ask the questions in *b*, *c*, and *d*.

107. c) The red lens is over the right eye, and the red lights appear to the left. Tell yourself that the lights have "crossed over," an idea to help you remember that this represents crossed diplopia. If the red lights were on the right, then they did not "cross over," and the diplopia would be uncrossed.

108. b) Crossed diplopia represents an exodeviation. (Think of the word "crossed" and a cross, or x.)

109. c) Stereopsis is measured in seconds of arc.

110. b) Bifoveal stereopsis is indicated when the patient can distinguish test items of less than 67 seconds of arc.

111. d) Twenty-five seconds of arc indicates finer stereo discrimination than 50 seconds of arc. Stereo vision is not measured in degrees of arc as given in answers *a* and *b*.

112. c) A patient with a constant ET or XT *over* 10 degrees will not have stereo vision. Nor will a monocular patient. A binocular patient with an intermittent deviation, phoria, or deviation of 10 degrees or less should have a stereo acuity test performed.

113. a) Stereopsis is present only in binocular individuals. Depth perception exists in binocular and monocular patients. Answers *b* and *c* are backwards: stereo vision involves seeing in three dimensions, and depth perception involves judging spatial relationships. Stereopsis is not learned; depth perception is.

114. c) Having the patient touch one pencil point to another is an indicator of gross stereopsis. (Try it on yourself: once with both eyes opened and once with one eye closed.) The Hirschberg estimates the size of a deviation, not stereopsis. Answers *b* and *d* are contrived.

115. a) Each of the tests listed utilized polarized glasses.

116. c) The fly was chosen as a test object because it is repulsive. An otherwise cooperative child may refuse to touch the fly because it is ugly and appears to be real. When the child sees it in 3-D, the huge fly seems to be standing on the page. Refusal is considered a positive indication that gross stereopsis exists.

117. b) Turning the test around 180 degrees will change the location of the stereo dots and make them appear sunken instead of elevated. If you turn the test 90 degrees it will not be stereopic. Polarized glasses are usually designed to be worn only one way. It is in the patient's best interest to get the most accurate measurement possible.

118. c) The raised dots of the Titmus test (at least the first three) can be guessed correctly by a nonfusing patient because the dots are off-center. The random dot E test offers no such clues. Neither test requires accurate color vision.

119. b) NPC is the point at which the eyes cannot maintain fusion on an object at near. The closer an object is to the eyes, the more convergence is required to fuse. Eventually fusion is no longer possible and breaks down, one eye drifting out.

120. c) NPC is measured objectively by bringing a small test object closer, usually alongside a ruler, and observing when fusion breaks and one eye drifts outward. Bringing an object closer and asking the patient to report diplopia is a subjective test for NPC. However, if a patient is suppressing, he will not notice the extra image when fusion breaks. Because of this, the examiner must watch for one eye to drift out in these cases. An amblyopic or monocular patient cannot do the subjective NPC because he does not have fusion. Accommodation does not contaminate the NPC measurement.

121. d) Of the items listed, only fusion is required. (A monocular patient, who has no fusion, will still have depth perception.)

122. b) NPC is more remote in adults. Children may measure from 5 to 10 cm, but adults may be more remote than 10 cm, and it tends to move further back with age. Patients with convergence insufficiency may have an NPC even greater than 25 cm. The test can be done objectively or subjectively (see question 120).

123. d) NPA measures the amount of accommodation, in diopters, that a patient has available for near viewing. It is not a measurement of the bifocal add. Answer *b* relates to NPC.

124. a) To test NPA, bring small print (J3, for example) closer to the patient until the patient reports that the letters have blurred.

125. b) Normally the patient (whether hyperopic or myopic) should wear full distance correction for the test. If the patient is too presbyopic to be able to see the test object from arm's length, you may test with her bifocals and subtract the add from the test result. Another option is to fully correct at distance and use a +2.50 lens over this, then subtract 2.50 from the test result. Every patient does not need a +2.50 lens, however; only those who are too presbyopic to test otherwise.

126. b) NPA should be checked in each eye. Fusion and depth perception are not required.

127. b) To convert distance to diopters, first get the distance in cm. Then divide the cm into 100. In this case, 100/12 cm = ~8.00 diopters.

128. a) First, find the diopters of accommodation with the glasses on: 100/28.5 = ~3.50. Now subtract the diopters provided by the glasses: 3.50 - 2.50 = 1.00 diopter.

129. b) Ductions refer to movements of one eye. Muscles that work against each other in the same eye are antagonists. Movements of both eyes in the same direction are versions. Movements of both eyes in opposite directions are vergences.

130. a) Testing ductions is useful when one eye is a fault for a deviation, as in restrictive strabismus. In answers *b* through *d* it would be more helpful to test versions.

131. d) Yoked muscles are muscles in both eyes that act to move the eyes in the same direction (ie, versions rather than ductions). For example, the RMR is yoked to the LLR for left gaze. The other answers are in the same eye (see question 129). The agonist is the muscle in one eye that is the primary mover for a given gaze.

132. c) Versions move both eyes in the same direction. Fusion does not necessarily occur; for example, the muscles in a blind eye are still innervated and linked to those of the other (seeing) eye.

133. a) Versions evaluate the function of yoked muscles. The other items are monocular.

134. c) Divergence is when the eyes move in opposite directions, away from each other. In versions, the eyes are moving together in the same direction.

135. b) Testing in head tilt position is done to test vertical deviations. Accommodative deviations and A/V patterns are associated with horizontal deviations.

136. d) The prism should be tilted with the head; that is, the bottom edge of the prism should be parallel to the floor of the orbit.

137. c) With head tilt right, the eyes will compensate to remain upright by intorting OD and extorting OS. The muscles that intort OD are RSR and RSO. The muscles that extort OS are LIO and LIR.

138. b) In the Bielschowsky head tilt test, hypertropia is evaluated first in head tilt right and then in head tilt left. Head tilt tests are not for horizontal deviations. See questions 41-46.

139. d) In most cases where the patient has developed a head tilt to compensate for a muscle deviation, the muscles involved are the obliques.

140. b) The rule in head tilts, turns, and tucks is that the head ends up *facing* the field of gaze where the *maximum* deviation is. This puts the eyes in the *opposite* direction where the deviation is *less*. Moving the head into the opposite position will often bring out the maximum deviation, perhaps rendering it observable.

141. b) The RSO is tested in down left gaze, which is where the primary problem will be in an RSO palsy. Tilting the head left and down puts the eye up and right, where the deviation is less.

142. b) Vergence is the ability of the eyes to fuse on the same object, whether it is close or far away, by moving the eyes inward or outward (that is, in the opposite direction). There may or may not be stereopsis. Versions move the eyes in the same direction; depth perception is judging spatial relationships.

143. b) As the object (mail truck) gets farther away, the eyes diverge until the point where the object is at infinity and the eyes are parallel.

144. a) Convergence is linked to accommodation. (Remember the "accommodative reflex" of accommodation, convergence, and miosis?)

145. d) When measuring fusional amplitudes, measure convergence last. Convergence is so strong that it can contaminate later measurements that require convergence to be relaxed. Because convergence is linked to near vision, distant testing should be done before near testing. So the proper order is: divergence distance, divergence near, convergence distance, convergence near.

146. d) To test divergence, place the prism with the base in. The eye will have to diverge to compensate. Convergence is tested with prism base out.

147. c) The break point of vergence is measured when the patient can no longer fuse and sees two images.

148. a) When the patient reports breaking, ask if he can pull the images together. If yes, move to the next strongest prism. If no, then you have indeed reached the break point. If the break point really is 20 diopters, then the images will be doubled with a 25 diopter (or any stronger) prism as well. Closing one eye will break fusion and invalidate the test.

149. c) Once the breaking point is recorded, you want to know the recovery point. This is found by introducing weaker and weaker prism until the images are fused again.

150. d) The power of a Risley prism is controlled by turning a small thumbscrew.

151. b) Using the Risley prism is convenient because you don't have a break as you put one prism down and pick another up, or a "line" as between prisms in a bar. There is a slow, continuous "slide" of power.

152. b) The red glass test can be used in all of the diagnostic positions of gaze. It is useless in cyclodeviations. Vertical as well as horizontal deviations can be measured.

153. a) A patient who is fusing will see a pink light or alternately, a blended red and white light. If only a white light is seen, then the eye behind the filter is suppressing. If only a red light is seen, then the other eye is suppressing. If two lights are seen, diplopia is present, indicating that fusion has been broken or does not exist.

154. b) The eye behind the filter (OS) is suppressing.

155. c) The red filter is over OD and the red light is on the right, indicating uncrossed diplopia. This signals that an esodeviation exists, so base out prism is used to neutralize. The endpoint is superimposition of the red and white lights.

156. c) NRC occurs when the fovea of each eye is receiving the same image and the brain can blend the images. A patient with a constant deviation cannot be using the foveae simultaneously.

157. a) ARC (also called anomalous retinal correspondence) sometimes occurs as an adaptation to untreated strabismus. The fovea of one eye corresponds to a nonfoveal point in the other eye. This sometimes allows some degree of fusion and vague stereopsis. Suppression and amblyopia may or may not be present as well.

158. c) Gross fusion does exist in ARC. Depth perception does exist (a monocular person has depth perception). There is no fine stereo acuity, and accommodation is not a factor.

159. b) See question 157. Although a nonretinal point is used, the brain is able to grossly fuse the images.

160. b) The Bagolini lenses are almost clear, so they hardly disrupt fusion, which is a distinct advantage. The test requires the Bagolini glasses or lenses. Its purpose is to evaluate fusion and retinal correspondence, not to differentiate between a phoria and a tropia. It is a subjective test, and cannot be done on infants.

161. a) The Bagolini lenses are placed one at axis 135 and one at axis 045. The key is for the axes to be 90 degrees from each other; 045 and 135 are conventional.

162. c) If the patient has trouble describing what she sees, have her draw the pattern. Normally two lines are seen, so asking if the line is on the left or right is of no import. If only one line is seen, however, you should ask in what direction the line slants. The test does not require normal color vision.

163. c) Seeing a cross indicates that fusion is present. If fusion occurs in an orthophoric patient, that patient is considered to have NRC.

164. c) Again, fusion is present. But so is a deviation. This indicates ARC.

165. d) A patient with ARC and suppression will report a solid line crossed by a line with a gap.

166. a) A patient who sees a single line is suppressing and does not have binocular vision. Seeing two lines that do not cross is considered a diplopic response with NRC.

Chapter 4. Visual Fields

1. d) Each mm on the retina equals 5 degrees on the visual field.

2. b) The rods and cones are the retina's light receptor cells. The retinal pigment epithelium is a retinal layer that lies *under* the rods and cones. The bipolar cells and ganglion cells are transmitters, not receptors.

3. c) An object on the patient's right will stimulate the temporal retina of the left eye and the nasal retina of the right eye. The foveae (plural of fovea) are used during central fixation, not for peripheral vision.

4. b) The nerve fibers are actually the axons of the ganglion cells.

5. Labeling (Figure 4-1):
   Horizontal raphe   d
   Temporal fibers   c
   Optic disc   a
   Radiating nasal fibers   b

6. Labeling (Figure 4-2):
   Superior retinal nerve fibers   f
   Optic disc   g
   Temporal retinal nerve fibers   a
   Macula   d
   Nasal retinal nerve fibers   e
   Horizontal raphe   b
   Inferior retinal nerve fibers   c

7. c) Because the nerve fibers fan out in a specific anatomic pattern, visual field defects occurring in the nerve fibers also follow the same pattern. This makes diagnosis easier because the patterns are identifiable.

8. c) The optic disc has no rods or cones to receive light impulses. It is therefore an area of blindness commonly called the "blind spot." The macula and fovea are at the center of the visual field, and are normally the areas of highest sensitivity. The lamina cribrosa is a sieve-like structure where the optic nerve goes through the sclera.

9. a) The average blind spot is 5.5 degrees wide and 7.5 degrees high.

10. d) The average blind spot is located 15 degrees temporal to fixation. (The optic disc is anatomically located in the nasal part of the retina, which picks up the temporal field.)

11. c) If you increase the test distance, the size of the blind spot increases in cm, but not in degrees. The size of the average blind spot is 5.5 x 7.5 degrees, regardless of test distance. However, at 1 m the blind spot is 9 x 13 cm; at 2 m the blind spot is 18 x 26 cm. This occurs because the size of the spot expands as you get further away, but the degree stays the same (like a cone).

12. c) At the chiasm, the nasal nerve fibers from each eye cross over to the other side. The temporal nerve fibers do not cross, but remain on the same side.

13. b) The pituitary gland lies just under the chiasm where the nasal fibers cross. If the pituitary swells, it can put pressure on the chiasm. This affects the crossing nasal fibers that receive impulses from the temporal field, producing a bitemporal field defect.

14. a) See question 13. The fibers that cross at the chiasm are more likely to be damaged in this scenario, thus the bitemporal hemianopsia is the most common. This type of loss affects the right field of vision in the right eye and the left field of vision in the left eye. *Note*: The terms *hemianopsia* and *hemianopia* are interchangeable.

15. b) After the chiasm, the nerve fibers continue on through the optic tract.

16. b) The nerve fibers rotate or twist as they pass through the optic tract.

17. d) The optic tract ends in the lateral geniculate body, which acts as a gathering place and relay station for the nerve fibers.

18. b) The lateral geniculate body has six layers; three are crossed and three are uncrossed.

19. a) The nerve fibers fan out into the optic radiations, enter the brain tissue, and are no longer contained or rotated within a tract. The temporal lobe fibers arch to form Meyer's loop.

20. b) The visual nerve fibers terminate into the occipital cortex of the brain. The eye-related fibers that terminate in the brain stem (only 10% of all the fibers) are concerned with pupillary action, and are not visual.

21. d) The closer a lesion is to the occipital lobe, the more congruous the visual field defects. This means that the field defect in one eye is more similar to the defect in the other. This phenomenon occurs because the fibers that correspond to neighboring visual spaces get closer and closer together as they course back to the occipital lobe.

22. d) An object on the patient's left will stimulate the nasal retina OS and temporal retina OD. The nasal fibers from OS will cross over to the right at the chiasm, while the temporal fibers from OD will remain on the right. These fibers stay on the right as they pass through the right optic tract, right lateral geniculate body, right optic radiations, and right occipital cortex.

23. a) An isopter is a boundary created around an area of the visual field that responds to the same stimulus.

24. d) A scotoma is an area within an isopter where vision is impaired or absent. The definition given (ie, no response to any stimulus on that particular machine) actually refers to an absolute scotoma. Bjerrum's is a particular type of scotoma that extends from the blind spot/optic nerve.

25. b) Threshold refers to a response to a stimulus, in a given area, 50% of the time.

26. c) An apostilb is a measurement of light intensity. It is not related to size (a large or small target may have the same brightness or intensity).

27. a) The decibel unit is used in automated perimetry.

28. a) The decibel unit is arbitrary because it can vary from one instrument to another, depending on the instrument's available maximum intensity.

29. a) See question 28.

30. c) The decibel unit represents a measurement of how much the maximum stimulus was *dimmed* before threshold was reached. Thus, the higher the decibel reading, the dimmer the target.

31. b) In Goldmann visual field testing, calibration is done prior to testing by checking and adjusting the projector light. Automated field instruments are generally self-calibrating, performing this task when first turned on.

32. Matching:

A. Absolute	i	
B. Altitudinal	o	
C. Bjerrum area	n	
D. Congruous	t	
E. Constricted	k	
F. Depression	l	
G. Eccentricities	b	
H. Fixation	a	
I. Hemianopsia	p	
J. Heteronymous	r	
K. Homonymous	s	
L. Incongruous	u	
M. Infrathreshold	e	
N. Isopter	g	
O. Meridians	c	
P. Quadrantanopsia	q	
Q. Relative	j	
R. Scotoma	h	
S. Step	m	
T. Suprathreshold	f	
U. Threshold	d	

33. b) Vision beyond fixation is the visual field. Binocular field is the visual field with both eyes. A neurological field is a particular method of testing. The visual pathway refers to the ocular structures responsible for sight.

34. d) The normal visual field is approximately 95 degrees temporal, 75 degrees inferior, 60 degrees nasal, and 60 degrees superior. You could pick this out even if the numbers were slightly different, if you remember that the temporal field is the largest and the nasal and superior fields are the smallest.

35. b) The superior and nasal fields are limited by the anatomical boundaries of the brow and nose. (The superior field also is limited by the lids, which are not mentioned in this question.)

36. b) The island of vision profile is a three-dimensional representation of the visual field. An isopter is a boundary. Comparative analysis and threshold graytone analysis are automated perimetry programs.

37. d) The peak of the island represents the area of highest visual sensitivity, the fovea.

38. a) The blind spot is devoid of light receptor cells, and would be represented by a bottomless hole. A peak is the point of highest sensitivity. A dip and a pit have a bottom, indicating that a stimulus could be found to which that area would respond.

39. a) The island of vision is afloat in a sea of blindness, because anything that is not seen is in a blind area. (The time-space continuum is a term I borrowed from Star Trek.)

40. b) Gradually decreasing vision would be represented by a gradually decreasing slope. A bottomless hole is a place of absolutely no vision. A sharp drop-off would be produced by an area where seeing suddenly becomes nonseeing. A flat area would be the same throughout, no increase or decrease.

41. c) The main purpose of screening techniques is to give a yes/no answer to the question: Is this patient's peripheral vision grossly normal? In general, screening techniques are quicker, and practical for evaluating large groups of people. (Not all at once, of course!) They also are useful in comparing a patient's screening results from one test to the next.

42. d) The screening protocol should vary according to the patient's presumed diagnosis. By the nature of the screening, the information obtained is not thorough; some defects will be missed.

43. a) The Harrington-Flocks screener uses a set of 10 cards, each with a central fixation dot. Each card has a different pattern that is visible only when an ultraviolet light is flashed on. After the flash, the patient describes the pattern that was seen. This tests several points at the same time (ie, multiple stimuli are used).

44. a) An automated field single intensity screening program first determines the threshold for several preselected points. From the patient's responses, the machine then builds (or extrapolates) a logical island of vision for that patient. The program then proceeds to screen other points using suprathreshold stimuli. This technique is okay for screening, but can miss defects that are just barely below suprathreshold.

45. b) While automated screening gives a yes/no response, automated threshold testing gives a value of threshold to each point that is tested. The illumination of the stimulus is individualized to each patient's responses.

46. d) In determining threshold (whether manual or automated), a point is tested numerous times. Starting with expected normal for a particular point is all right, but is not required. Testing a point only once would be single intensity screening.

47. a) A suprathreshold stimulus is not seen 100% of the time, but rather is considered to be seen only 95% of the time. It is extrapolated that suprathreshold could be missed 5% of the time, in part by chance alone.

48. b) Since kinetic perimetry involves a moving target, the patient is responding to movement as well as size and intensity.

49. d) Automated threshold tests usually start with suprathreshold, decrease intensity until the light is not seen, then increase again to confirm the reading. In manual threshold, it is customary to start infrathreshold and increase intensity until the target is seen.

50. c) The optic nerve has no threshold because it cannot perceive any light stimulus.

51. b) The validity of any type of field testing depends on the patient's ability and willingness to maintain fixation. Automated perimetry requires minimal technical skill as compared to the manual Goldmann. Other factors involved (but not listed as responses) are the patient's response time, vision, and mental capabilities.

52. c) The blind spot cannot be plotted on the Amsler grid because it falls outside of the grid's testing range of the central 20 degrees.

53. b) Because of poor vision, many low vision patients have difficulty seeing the fixation area and maintaining fixation on it. For tangent screen testing, a large X of white tape can be placed over the fixation button. Many automated perimeters have an alternate fixation area made up of several lights instead of just one, that may be used in low vision testing situations.

54. d) Manual perimetry, from confrontation to Goldmann, involves moving and stationary targets. Theoretically, any and every point could be tested, not merely preselected ones.

55. b) See question 54. Automated perimetry uses preselected points, is more accurate with static threshold testing, and is more reproducible.

56. c) It is a disadvantage that manual visual field testing, as with the Goldmann perimeter, requires more technical skill than automated.

57. c) In confrontation visual field testing, the assumption is that the examiner's visual field is normal. A technician with an abnormal field cannot perform accurate confrontation fields. The patient need not have 20/20 vision. The peripheral area, rather than the central area, is tested. The test is not qualitative.

58. c) The advantage of the confrontation field is that it requires no equipment and can be performed on a patient in any position (ie, sitting or lying down). Properly done, the test will pick up gross defects. Most school-aged children can cooperate for a confrontation field test.

59. b) While the examiner's fingers most often are used as the target, one also may use objects such as a dropper bottle lid. The other statements are true.

60. b) The central 30 degrees are mapped on the tangent screen or Autoplot®.

61. d) The Autoplot® must be used at a 1 m test distance.

62. c) The patient's responses should be marked with black-headed pins if using a felt screen. The nap would be ruined when trying to erase chalk or pencil marks. Shiny sewing pin heads could distract the patient.

63. a) The patient should wear his habitual distance correction when taking the tangent screen test.

64. b) The patient should tuck her head to lower the bifocal add out of the way when testing the lower portion of the field. Make sure she maintains fixation, however. Using the bifocal for the inferior field would invalidate the test, since the upper half would be tested with one correction and the lower half in another.

65. a) Stand on the patient's left when plotting the left and on the right when plotting the right. Don't reach across the screen with the wand and target.

66. b) Move the target smoothly at about 5 degrees per second.

67. a) "2/1000 green" refers to a 2 mm test object, a test distance of 1000 mm (which equals 1 m), and a green test object.

68. b) Most tangent screens are 2 x 2 m, and the usual test distance is 1 m. In some situations (such as suspected malingering or hysteria), the patient might be moved back to a test distance of 2 m. There is a 4 x 4 m screen with a usual test distance of 2 m.

69. d) If doubling the test distance to catch a malingerer, you also should double the object size (in this case, to 6 mm). If, with this combination, the patient still plots the exact same isopter, you should strongly suspect malingering or hysteria.

70. c) An arc perimeter consists of an arc-shaped screen that is rotated according to which meridian is being tested. The target is moved manually or mechanically. The patient puts his chin in a chin rest.

71. a) Arc perimetry is most useful for kinetically plotting outer isopters.

72. b) To test the right eye, the chin goes in the left chin rest (and vice versa).

73. c) Habitual distance correction is worn during arc perimetry.

74. b) The Goldmann perimeter is bulky and not very portable at all.

75. c) Before proceeding with the field, determine a threshold point at about 25 degrees temporal to fixation. (Since glaucoma usually is what you are screening for, start with the near portion of the field, as most early glaucoma defects occur in the central 30 degrees.)

76. a) Use the smallest, dimmest stimulus that will give an isopter of proper dimensions. Adjust brightness (with Arabic numbered or alphabetic levers) before resorting to size (Roman numeral levers). In most cases, an "e" lever can be used, so this rarely is changed. Start with I (the smallest size) and 2e. Increase brightness by going to 3, then 4. If there is no response to I4e, increase the size by single steps until you get a response. If the patient's response doesn't make sense (based on the patient's vision, diagnosis, and ability), check the stimulus lever to be sure it is on (not off) when depressed. You also may need to re-educate the patient. Answer *b decreases* the stimulus size and brightness, which is the exact opposite of what you need to do. Answer *c increases* stimulus size immediately, also not the correct progression in this case. Answer *d* is not too far off the mark, because intensity increases before size, but the starting point is too low. The I2a is the smallest and almost dimmest stimulus available. Starting with the I2e requires less trial and error, less time, and less fatigue (for both patient and examiner). See also questions 77 to 79 and 82, which deal with stimulus selection.

77. d) See question 76. 4e is the brightest target, so if the patient doesn't respond to it, the target *size* must be increased.

78. d) The normal field extends to 95 degrees temporally. Central is 30 degrees. To map the outer isopter, use a target that is threshold between 30 and 95, or around 50 degrees temporal to fixation. A target that is threshold at fixation or 30 degrees would be too dim to map the outer periphery. At 15 degrees temporal, you run into the blind spot.

79. b) When performing a follow-up test, use the same stimuli as the original test. This provides better comparisons. If changes have occurred, you may have to plot additional isopters/points using other stimuli as well.

80. a) If the patient has trouble seeing the central fixation area, use the mirror in the viewing port. You either can flash it manually during testing, or just flip it down and leave it in place (after determining that fixation will be adequate, since the eye no longer can be seen through the telescope). An add for the whole test will not give an accurate outer field, nor will the patient's glasses. Never tape anything to the inside of the bowl, as this will mar the paint finish.

81. c) Central fields are within 30 degrees.

82. c) To map the central field, use a stimulus that is threshold at 25 degrees temporal to fixation. The threshold stimulus at central fixation would be too dim to test the central field. The blind spot is at the 15 degrees temporal point. It may be that the proper stimulus is two notches dimmer than that used for the outer isopter, but you must test to find out.

83. a) Move the stimulus at a steady pace about 5 degrees per second. If you oscillate the target, it effectively becomes larger (which makes it easier to see). Isopters are measured along meridians, not eccentricities.

84. b) Isopters and scotomas are mapped by moving the stimulus from an area where it is not seen to an area where it is seen (and the patient responds). A stationary stimulus is not used to plot borders. Moving the stimulus from left to right is useful only when plotting the 180 degree meridian.

85. b) Enlargement of the blind spot should make it easier to find, not more difficult. The other answers are common errors.

86. c) To map at 90 and 180 degrees, plot meridians 5 and 15 degrees to either side. Plotting exactly at 90 or 180 might cause you to miss a step defect. In addition, the Goldmann bowl itself has a gap at 180 and 0 degrees, so the patient's true response might be missed because the stimulus is not actually being projected.

87. b) A defect should be mapped with at least two different stimuli. A test strategy is necessary, but the strategy must be modified as you accommodate every patient. An add is not used for fields beyond the central 30 degrees, and a +3.00 is not right for every patient.

88. c) The patient has shown a decrease of 30 degrees in a 25 degree meridian change. The field should be more round than this, if it is normal. You simply cannot discount the abnormality by automatically connecting the points. Plot a new point by moving the stimulus perpendicular to an imaginary line connecting the two points. This will give a more accurate picture than plotting along an intermediate meridian. Using a brighter or larger stimulus will move the point out on the 150 degree meridian, but it also will move the point out on the 175 degree meridian.

89. a) Monitoring fixation on the Goldmann perimeter can be done constantly by looking through the viewer port. Unfortunately, the fixation mirror obstructs the view. If you need to use the mirror you can flash it by hand, or move it every now and then to check the patient's position. Many automated perimeters check fixation by flashing a light on the blind spot. If the patient responds, it is recorded as a fixation loss. A manual field on a cooperative patient takes about 12 minutes; checking fixation once every 5 minutes is not enough.

90. c) Automated tests may include any number of points.

91. b) If the pupil is smaller than 3 mm, consider dilating the patient before proceeding with the test.

92. Matching:
    A. Back up   g
    B. Default   h
    C. Field   c
    D. Formatting   f
    E. Keyboard   b
    F. Menu   d
    G. Monitor   a
    H. Parameters   j
    I. Point array   i
    J. Return or enter key   e

93. b) Initializing or formatting a disk erases *all* of the information on it. You never will initialize the hard drive. This not only would erase data files but program files as well.

94. a) Most automated perimeters present the target for 0.1 to 0.4 seconds.

95. c) Stereopsis is a binocular phenomenon. Visual fields testing is monocular. The intensity of the background and stimulus affects threshold, in that a dimmer background increases contrast and a brighter stimulus is easier to see. Threshold decreases with age and with distance from the fovea.

96. a) A dimmer background means that the stimulus will show up more because contrast is increased.

97. a) Most automated perimeters have an alternate fixation pattern that can be used for low-vision patients. This pattern is offset from normal fixation, hence the term *eccentric*. If the eccentric fixation pattern is activated, the instrument automatically adjusts the blind spot and other points to coincide. Turning off the fixation monitor won't help the patient see the fixation point any better, nor will using a larger target. The correcting lens must be calculated for each patient; a +3.00 lens used across the board is unacceptable.

98. a) The automated field machine compares the patient's responses to that of normal individuals. If the patient's response falls outside the 95th, it is considered abnormal.

99. b) Normal for a screening test does not necessarily mean that there is no field loss. It means that there is no field loss detected at this time by this particular instrument and this particular test. Screening programs can miss the shallow defects that indicate the early stages of disease. The need for future formal visual field tests depends on the patient's diagnosis and complaints. Screening tests are not adequate in glaucoma evaluation. Diagnosis of glaucoma requires elevated pressures and nerve damage, in addition to field loss.

100. b) One of the beauties of automated perimetry is that it is largely independent of operator bias and expertise.

101. b) Automated perimeters differ in the intensity of their backgrounds and stimuli. These intensities affect the outcome of the test, so when comparing a field from one instrument to another, read the scale values carefully. It is true that some instruments use projection and others use LEDs, but this is not a primary factor in comparing fields. The correcting lens for the same patient on the same day may vary from one instrument to another, depending on the distance from the patient to the screen. The correcting lens must be calculated and used for the central 30 degrees, regardless of the instrument used.

102. b) Bringing a target from nonseeing into seeing until the patient responds is kinetic perimetry. (The word *kinetic* refers to motion or movement.) Static perimetry involves a stationary target, as does threshold. Formal perimetry usually refers to Goldmann or computer-generated visual fields (as opposed to confrontation, for example).

103. a) See question 102. Automated perimetry means that the test was computerized, not necessarily how the test was done. While threshold perimetry does use stationary targets, the term generally refers to finding the smallest, dimmest target that a receptor can detect. (That qualification was not mentioned in this question.)

104. a) Automated perimeters most often use static perimetry, although a few can do kinetic perimetry with the right software. True, automated perimeters usually use decibel designations, but that is a unit of measurement, not a testing technique.

105. b) The Harrington-Flocks cannot be changed to incorporate moving targets.

106. d) Since threshold testing is a matter of finding the dimmest and smallest target that the receptor can detect, it is a function of contrast sensitivity.

107. a) Mapping isopters with kinetic perimetry is like mapping the island of vision as if you are floating above it.

108. d) Answers *a*, *b*, and *c* are descriptions of kinetic isopter mapping. Static perimetry is like dropping a paratrooper from above onto one single, selected spot, and measuring how far down the trooper fell to reach the ground.

109. b) Threshold static perimetry is the most sensitive of the tests listed. Suprathreshold static testing presents a single stimulus that "should be" seen based on an extrapolated hill of vision for that patient. Because a moving target is easier to see than a stationary one, kinetic testing of any kind is less sensitive.

110. c) The bulb of the Goldmann perimeter should be calibrated once a day. The background should be adjusted for every patient with the patient seated at the instrument, because various clothing materials and colors reflect and absorb light in differing amounts.

111. c) The maximum light projected by the Goldmann is 1000 asbs. (However, it is possible to increase the equivalent value to 100,000 asbs by increasing the size of the stimulus.)

112. a) The correct background illumination is 31.5 asbs.

113. d) To calibrate the stimulus, the levers are set at V4e.

114. d) If the stimulus is not 1000 asbs, you might try rotating the bulb 180 degrees and measure again. If that doesn't work, then replacing the bulb is the only option. If the fuse is out the machine won't light at all. You should not compensate by readjusting the background light.

115. c) The levers should be at V1e when you set the background illumination. This makes the stimulus measure 31.5 asbs, the same as the illumination desired for the background.

116. a) Slide the bulb shield until the luminescence of the bowl equals that of the target. You can't count on the imprinted scale to be accurate.

117. d) Check the printer paper supply each day before beginning. Automated perimeters are self-calibrating and run their own internal diagnostic without any prompting, so *a - c* aren't necessary.

118. b) If you see threshold values other than <0, it is time to change the bulb. The instrument still can be turned on, and it still can find the blind spot. Unexplained field contraction is not related to the bulb.

119. d) The visual field test is a subjective test, not objective. Any response from a patient is always subjective; objective tests do not require patient response.

120. b) The Goldmann field chart traditionally is hand-marked with colored pencils. Each color corresponds to a different stimulus size and intensity, and is coded to the chart at the lower right corner of the chart. Checks and x's in lead pencil would be hard to decode. Grayscale printouts are products of automated fields. There is no pantograph.

121. c) Areas of inconsistency can be marked with a crosshatch and labeled "in and out" or "variable." Such an area cannot be plotted as if it had definite borders. Moving the target faster would make the area map as smaller (or even cause it to disappear), but it would be a false response. The same speed should be used throughout the test. Ignoring such a finding is likewise incorrect.

122. d) Static spot-checking can be indicated by a small colored mark on the chart. Isopters are plotted using kinetic testing, not static. Coloring in that entire part of the grid would be misleading, since theoretically there are an almost infinite number of points within any area.

123. d) Data must be entered the same way every time. If you enter *Charles James* for one test and *James Charles* for the next, the computer will not know they are the same patient. Data from a previous test needs to be updated. For example, pupil size or near add prescription might have changed. The computer only knows what you tell it. Data is lost if the instrument is turned off before the information is saved.

124. b) Floppy disks should be removed from the instrument before the computer is turned off.

125. c) The decibel values corresponding to the point where the number is printed on the chart is characteristic of the numeric pattern (also called the value table) printout style. In addition, the numbers represent retinal sensitivity. A "0" means that the brightest stimulus was shown and not seen. Lower numbers indicate brighter lights, and are more commonly elicited in the periphery. The higher numbers around the fovea represent dimmer lights and greater retinal sensitivity. Numbers are used, not symbols. The numbers are the actual values, and represent "truth;" that is, the numbers are not statistically altered in any way. Decibels are given, not apostilbs.

126. d) See question 125.

127. a) The grayscale printout gives each decibel measurement a graphic symbol, then prints the field using the symbols. The symbols used are varying shades of gray. The darker the symbol, the higher the decibel and the less sensitive the receptors.

128. c) A point that is not seen would appear as a black area on the grayscale printout.

129. c) The best grayscale printout would accompany a comprehensive threshold test. The suprathreshold single stimulus test and the hill of vision profile do not use a grayscale. The three-zone test uses three or four symbols, not the broader array as in a full grayscale.

130. a) The depth of defect printout is an analysis that compares the patient's actual threshold values to the threshold values that were expected. The numbers are printed at the corresponding point locations. (It does not compare the patient to normal patients.) It does not give actual decibels or apostilbs.

131. c) The comparison printout is designed to compare a patient's previous test to the present test.

132. b) A -2 on a comparison printout means that the patient has lost 2 decibels (at that particular point) since the previous test.

133. d) The need for a correcting lens is determined on a patient-by-patient basis. A 50-year-old who is -2.50 sphere will probably not require a near add. A 20-year-old who wears +6.00 sphere will need an add. (The words "every" and "only" should have clued you in that answers *b* and *c* were wrong.)

134. b) The central 30 degrees is the testing area where a near add is required. True, the fovea and blind spot are within this area, but answer *b* is the best because it includes both.

135. d) A lens with a thin rim is the best type of trial lens to use. The patient's glasses, or a trial lens with a thick rim, most likely will cause artificial field losses because the edge of the lens or the rim will block off part of the patient's side vision. Cylinder power cannot be ignored, either (see question 139).

136. b) Visual field landmarks will be displaced if the distance correction is over +10.00. (See questions 137 and 138 as well.) The use of a contact lens is desirable, but not required. A trial lens never is used for the entire test as long as some stimulus can be detected outside the central 30 degrees.

137. a) A high hyperope will exhibit a compressed field with a blind spot displaced closer to fixation than normal.

138. b) By contrast, a high myope will have an expanded field with a blind spot farther away from fixation than normal.

139. d) Cylinder is translated to a spherical equivalent if the amount is under 1.00 diopter. If over 1.00 diopter, the full correction is used.

140. c) An emmetropic patient between the ages of 30 and 40 is given a near correcting lens (+1.00 sphere).

141. c) The near add calculation starts with the patient's distance refractometric measurement and then incorporates an add related to the patient's age. The habitual near add cannot be used because it may not be set to the 300 mm test distance of the Goldmann and some automated instruments.

142. d) A +3.25 add is required for a fully dilated patient, regardless of age.

143. c) In automated perimetry, the near add calculation must include the patient's full distance correction, an age-related add, and the bowl depth. Bowl depth can range from 30 cm (equal to a Goldmann perimeter) to 50 cm. Most computerized perimeters calculate the add for you once you input the distance Rx and patient age.

144. a) The near add should be placed with the sphere closest to the patient's eye (if cylinder is also required) and as close to the patient's eye as possible. Vertex distance is not usually considered when going from glasses to trial lens.

145. c) Vertex distance is important, however, when calculating a contact lens to use. While this example does not include vertex distance or a conversion chart, logical deduction should lead to the correct answer. First, the question states that the contact is for the outer field, so you can discount the +3.00 add; this indicates that answers *c* and *d* are incorrect. It takes more plus power to do the same job as the lens gets closer to the eye. Thus, +11.00 is the best answer offered.

146. c) The Roman numeral levers control the size of the stimulus.

147. b) The Arabic number and alphabetic levers control the intensity of the stimulus. The numbers designate 0.5 log unit steps (4 being the brightest), and the letters designate 0.1 log unit steps (e being the brightest).

148. c) In the case of extreme low vision, try starting with the V4e, which is the largest and brightest stimulus. (There is no such thing as a VI6f setting.)

149. b) Performing a confrontation field on the patient prior to formal perimetry serves to reinforce the idea that "you will not be looking directly at the target" and "you need to look straight ahead during the entire test." Confrontation fields will not give you a threshold, quantitate defects, or give visual acuity.

150. d) Ideally, an opaque white patch is used because it not only covers the untested eye, but keeps the eye light adapted. A black patch allows the eye to become dark adapted. (A person can be dark adapted in one eye and light adapted in the other.)

151. c) Patients should be told *not* to look at the stimulus. Telling patients that they won't see every light right away reduces a lot of stress, because normally they think, "I must be doing terribly because I don't see anything." Tell them that they may go for a while without seeing anything. They also should know that they are to respond regardless of the size or brightness of the stimulus. Patients should respond as soon as they are aware of the light, and not wait for it to get crystal clear.

152. b) The eye should be level with the fixation area. It is okay if the patient has to lean forward a little as long as the back is straight and not hyperextended. The plane of the face should be parallel to the plane of the back of the bowl or screen. If the chin is jutted forward, this will minimize the lower field. If the forehead is jutted out, the size of the superior field is reduced.

153. b) Patients who cannot press the buzzer may turn the buzzer upside down and press the button into their knee, leg, armrest, or tabletop. Giving a verbal response or a nod will interfere with fixation and positioning.

154. a) A patient with the chin tucked down has a reduction of the superior field because of interference by the brow. You must visually check the head position, because it still is possible to align the eye and for the patient to fixate even if the head is malpositioned.

155. c) If a man has a full beard, have him put his chin beyond the chin rest, then slide back into the chin cup. Then the hair can be parted to either side of the chin cup so as not to interfere with the inferior field. A beard can cushion the chin in the cup, making it difficult to maintain alignment.

156. d) The patient's back should be straight, not hyperextended, even if he has to lean forward a little. Feet should be flat on the floor, thighs parallel to the floor.

157. a) Perching the wheelchair (or any) patient on a board for the test would be uncomfortable and probably dangerous. Remove parts of the wheelchair, if possible, in order to accommodate. If you remove the armrests, be sure the patient isn't going to fall out of the chair. Propping with pillows may help with comfort and positioning.

158. a) The longer the test continues, the greater the patient's fatigue, boredom, and "hypnosis." These all lower reliability. The test may stretch on because the program does not find that the data is reliable.

159. c) Give patients verbal encouragement. This helps them stay alert and motivated. For example, tell them they're doing well, or that they're halfway through, etc. Answer *a* might be considered correct by some. My opinion is that if you tell patients to hold down the button and pause whenever they want to, it will lengthen the test and add to the stress, instead of helping the patient. It is better to let pauses remain in the control of the perimetrist. Patients should not be allowed to sit at the machine with their eyes closed during the test. Resting every 5 minutes might be allowed in extreme cases, but not as a general rule.

160. d) The projector arm of the Goldmann swings around the patient. If a patient sits back unannounced, he could get clobbered. True, sitting back means the test takes longer, fixation is lost, and the patient must be repositioned. But *d* is the best answer because the test is not invalidated, nor is repositioning difficult (even if it is bothersome).

161. d) It is helpful to run a few test points to give the patient an idea of what the test is like before you begin plotting anything.

162. c) Burning, watery eyes are symptoms of dryness. In the case of a visual field exam, dryness usually is caused by staring. Before starting the test and sometime during the test, remind the patient to blink periodically. You can stop the test and instill artificial tear drops if necessary.

163. a) Communication during an automated field is almost constant. The droning of the machine and rhythm of responses can be tiring for even the most alert patients. Automated fields are taxing; therefore, reinforce the patient often. Leaving the room is not a good idea. Even the best patient can slip out of alignment.

164. b) The suprathreshold test finds a threshold point, then tests the entire field with a stimulus brighter than the threshold. This is equivalent to plotting a single isopter and finding deep scotomas. Shallow scotomas may be missed. There is no such thing as infrathreshold single stimulus testing (ie, testing only with an infrathreshold stimulus). Multiple stimulus testing uses both supra- and infrathreshold targets.

165. d) Because the single stimulus suprathreshold may not pick up early (shallow) defects, it is not suitable in glaucoma field testing. The three-zone is a screening technique. While not ideal for glaucoma, it does differentiate between absolute and relative scotomas. Tests in answers *b* and *c* are comprehensive enough for glaucoma evaluation.

166. b) The two-zone format is like the suprathreshold single stimulus above. The hill of vision profile is made up from threshold data. The three-zone format is like the two-zone, except that areas where the suprathreshold stimulus is not seen are checked with yet another stimulus in order to differentiate between relative and absolute scotomas. Bracketing (staircasing) is a method of detecting threshold, where the stimulus is made brighter if the patient misses it or dimmer if the patient sees it.

167. d) See question 166.

168. c) The quantify defects strategy actually determines threshold for points missed on suprathreshold testing. Three-zone determines whether a scotoma is relative or absolute, but does not give an actual threshold reading for the area.

169. d) Suprathreshold testing is a screening tool, not intended for glaucoma evaluation. Nor does the size of the pupil matter in this scenario.

170. a) In order for tests to be comparable, they must be run with the same parameters. Otherwise, you are trying to compare apples and stones. The correcting lens used for one test may not be appropriate for the next. The patient always should be instructed, even if she has done numerous field tests. It may be easier to manage files if they are on the same floppy disk, but this is not required.

171. b) Most automated field programs test points that are 6 degrees apart. Certain macular evaluations might test points that are 2 degrees apart, but they are not the most commonly used programs.

172. c) If looking for steps, it is best to straddle the horizontal and vertical meridians. (If you test directly on those meridians you might miss the defect.) The array should straddle the meridians by 2 or 3 degrees.

173. c) An array that is intended for glaucoma screening will emphasize Bjerrum's area, the blind spot, and the nasal meridian. Other optic nerve diseases may show up in the temporal area, which is not tested as closely on a glaucoma test.

174. b) If a defect is close to fixation (such as a defect found on an Amsler grid), choose an array that will test the central 10 degrees with more concentration, 2 degrees apart. Testing the entire field at 2 degree intervals would be very time-consuming. A red stimulus usually is used in neurological testing.

175. b) Running a threshold test that used starting points determined by a threshold point in each quadrant would be most appropriate in evaluating optic neuritis. This is because the field loss in optic neuritis can change rapidly. Thus, the results of a previous test may be drastically different from the current situation. The test would take longer as the program fumbles around trying to find threshold. The same is true of using age-related normals. A field performed at 2 dB higher than a previous test assumes that improvement greater than this is not possible; thus, this test isn't suitable either.

176. b) If, during threshold testing, it becomes obvious that the patient cannot physically cope with the testing time required, switch to a screening strategy. This will provide some information and won't take as long. Increasing the stimulus size might create an erroneous result. Education is not the problem here; endurance is.

177. b) Just knowing that you are watching will make the patient more motivated to hold fixation. A few Goldmann perimetrists advocate telling the patient where the next kinetic stimulus is coming from, but most perimetrists do not feel this is a good idea. Using the near add may clear the fixation target, but cannot be used to plot the outer isopter. The fixation point need be enlarged only for low vision patients. Fixation in a visually capable patient is a matter of will power.

178. Matching:
    A. Fixation loss   c,g,j
    B. False positive   a,d
    C. False negative   b,f
    D. Fluctuation   e,h,i

179. b) If the patient seems to be fixating, yet the instrument is registering fixation losses, tell the program to relocate the blind spot or reduce the fixation stimulus. If the blind spot is not placed accurately, the patient will respond when the light is flashed in that area. Reducing the intensity of the stimulus may help, as well.

180. a) An infrared monitor evaluates fixation via the corneal reflex in front of the pupil. The change from a black pupil to a blue iris is more pronounced than the change from a black pupil to a brown iris, hence fixation losses in a blue eye are registered more easily.

181. c) "Catch trials" refers to the methods used by automated perimetry programs to evaluate patient cooperation and performance. These include monitoring fixation losses, false positives, and false negatives.

182. a) The correcting lens should be in place when you are testing the central 30 degrees.

183. b) A patient with a slow response time will cause the isopters to be contracted artificially and the blind spot to be enlarged artificially. A larger or brighter stimulus triggers a response sooner than a smaller or dimmer stimulus. Moving the stimulus too slowly moves the isopters out by giving the patient more time to respond. Oscillating the stimulus has the effect of enlarging it.

184. a) The most common areas for visual field artifacts are superior nasal (because of brows and lids) and inferior nasal (because of the nose).

185. c) Using the wrong power lens can wreak havoc on the field, giving you some truly strange results. For one thing, minification or magnification might be a factor. Blurred vision might be another. In addition, placing the lens as close to the eye as possible reduces any interference by the lens rim (even a thin lens rim, which is the only type that should be used anyway). Using spherical correction is not proper if the patient has astigmatism over 1.00 diopter. The lens is used to test the field within the central 30 degrees, not beyond it.

186. a) The wrong correcting lens power also may cause a generalized depression of the field.

187. Matching:
Ptotic upper eyelid   b
Thick rim on correcting lens   d
Hysteria or malingering   a
Decentered correcting lens   c

188. a) Retinal defects are monocular. The remaining statements are true.

189. d) Retinal defects are projected to the opposite quadrant. Thus, superior is projected to inferior and nasal to temporal.

190. c) Since the macula is the area of fine central vision, any defect involving the macula will be more debilitating than a defect in any other area.

191. d) Nerve fiber layer damage causes field losses that follow along the nerve fiber pattern. Thus, Bjerrum's scotomas are the most common nerve fiber layer field loss listed. Hemianopsias, quadrantanopsias, and congruous defects generally occur posterior to the junction of the optic nerve and chiasm. (Retinal detachment is a possible exception.)

192. b) All nerve fibers lead to the disc. Thus, defects in the nerve fiber layer lead to the blind spot (not horizontally and not vertically). There is a definite pattern of progression.

193. d) A left homonymous hemianopsia would occur posterior to the chiasm, not involving the retinal fiber layer as in answers *a* through *c*.

194. c) Ocular hypertension has no field loss. The definition of ocular hypertension is IOP that is above normal but where no optic nerve damage or field loss occurs.

195. b) Retinal detachment causes a field loss that is projected to the opposite quadrant. It does not cause enlargement of the blind spot per se, as do the other answers.

196. c) Optic nerve disease other than glaucoma usually causes an enlargement of the blind spot that is more equal in all directions, producing a rounder (concentric) scotoma. In glaucoma, the nerve damage occurs more unequally, usually causing first vertical orientation, and later, horizontal.

197. c) The most common finding in optic nerve damage is a central scotoma. This is because the nerve fibers from the macula move to a central position about 1 cm behind the disc. Thus, any pressure on the disc would affect the macular fibers.

198. a) Optic nerve damage is monocular until the fibers reach the junction between the nerve and the chiasm. Thus, there is an area just anterior to the chiasm that will cause a binocular defect. In addition, the question specifies optic nerve damage. Anatomically, the optic nerve ceases to exist at the chiasm.

199. a) The field loss experienced in optic neuritis can resolve. In fact, about half of all patients with optic neuritis will have normal fields less than a year later. Answers *b* through *d* are true.

200. b) Optic disc drusen can cause a field defect that mimics glaucoma. The important difference is that the drusen nasal step is inferior, while the glaucomatous nasal step is superior.

201. d) The most common field defect seen in optic disc drusen is an inferior nasal step. Defects in answers *a* through *c* also can occur, but are less common.

202. d) Field loss in patients taking Plaquenil may include paracentral and pericentral scotomas as well as central scotoma. Infrequently, constriction may occur.

203. d) Due to the pattern of glaucoma damage to specific retinal nerve fibers, glaucoma classically causes changes in the nasal field (nasal step), central 20 degrees (Bjerrum's scotoma), and the blind spot (enlargement).

204. a) The time-honored method of glaucoma screening was developed by Drs. Armaly and Drance. This screening technique pays special attention to the areas listed in question 203.

205. c) The pattern of field loss in glaucoma directly corresponds to how the nerve fiber layers are being damaged. This is not related to the pressure, since a person can have elevated IOP and no damage, or normal IOP and experience a field loss. The damage is a result of the pressure on the optic disc, not the blood supply in the choroid. In addition, the damage is to the nerve fiber layer itself, not posterior into the visual pathway.

206. b) The nasal step in glaucoma is superior. It generally is not connected to the blind spot, as is a Bjerrum's scotoma.

207. c) Early glaucomatous defects include a paracentral scotoma in Bjerrum's area, and a nasal step. Answer *b* is correct, but answer *c* is more correct.

208. b) Bjerrum's area is in the 15 degree eccentricity.

209. d) In end-stage glaucoma, before total blindness occurs, there remains a temporal crescent of vision. At this point, even the typical glaucoma tunnel vision has been lost.

210. c) The more congruous a defect is, the more posterior it is located (as a general rule). Prechiasmal and optic nerve lesions are monocular, and hence not congruous.

211. a) Because of the anatomical location of the retinal nerve fibers, neurological lesions respect (ie, do not cross) the vertical meridian.

212. b) See question 211 above.

213. a) The optic nerve is prechiasmal, hence a defect would be monocular. A homonymous defect is, by definition, binocular.

214. c) Because the only place where the temporal fibers are together is the chiasm, the chiasm is the only place where a bitemporal defect can occur.

215. c) A wedge-shaped field loss is the "pie." A wedge in the upper quadrant ("in the sky") indicates that the fibers to the inferior retinas have been damaged. A wedge in the lower quadrant ("on the floor") indicates that fibers to the superior retinas have been damaged. These kinds of defects occur where the fibers fan out in the optic radiations.

216. c) Patients with migraines sometimes notice a shimmering area of blanked-out vision, or the vision will seem to close in with shimmering on the outer edges. This is known as a *visual aura*, and may signal that a headache is on the way. However, the visual disturbance also can occur without any headache (ophthalmic migraine).

217. d) Spiral, star-shaped, and tubular fields are all findings in the hysterical patient.

218. c) Hysteria is actually a neurosis, and usually is caused by mental conflict of some sort. A desire to trick the examiner is malingering. Elevated IOP and pseudotumor do not cause hysteria.

219. d) Nonexpanding (tubular) and spiral fields are more easily detected on the Goldmann or by tangent screen. Also, in these two tests, the examiner has the option of moving the patient back from the screen in order to retest.

220. a) A field loss pattern that cannot be reproduced from one testing to another is an indication of nonorganic field loss. Organic patterns generally will resemble each other from one exam to the next.

221. b) An enlarged blind spot is not a hallmark of nonorganic field loss. The other items are. Especially interesting (and tell-tale) is the fact that while visual acuity is reduced, foveal thresholds are measured at normal.

222. Matching:

Chiasmal defect	g
Glaucoma	f
Nerve fiber layer defect	d
Nonorganic defect	b
Optic disc drusen	e
Postchiasmal defect	c
Retinal detachment	a

Chapter 5. Contact Lenses

1. d) Because a PMMA lens is not oxygen permeable, nearly all PMMA lenses cause some degree of corneal anoxia (an = without, oxia = oxygen). This, in turn, is responsible for corneal warpage. Because gas permeable lenses *do* allow oxygen to reach the cornea, the incidence (and risk) of corneal warpage is much less. In the absence of corneal complications, either rigid lens should provide crisp vision, are equally easy to handle, and can be ground to correct astigmatism.

2. a) PMMA lenses are still used in cases of high astigmatism, such as keratoconus. Because of the thickness of a high plus or minus lens, they generally are not recommended for high refractive errors. Presbyopia is better corrected with gas permeable or soft lenses.

3. a) Ectatic corneal dystrophy is another name for keratoconus. If corneal anesthesia exists, the patient might damage the cornea with the lens because the lens can't be felt. Because the position and movement of a hard lens depends on the lids, patients with lid problems (malformations, scarring, etc.) are not good candidates. A patient with dry eye is not a good candidate either, because the cornea depends entirely on the tear film for oxygen.

4. b) PMMA is not oxygen permeable.

5. c) Because PMMA is not oxygen permeable, most PMMA wearers have some degree of corneal anoxia (see question 1).

6. b) The soft lens is hydrophilic, which means "loves water." The fact that it absorbs water is responsible for its entire nature. This includes comfort, flexibility, oxygen transmission, etc. There is very little tear exchange under a soft lens (as opposed to a rigid lens). These lenses are not resistant to deposits. A larger diameter is possible because of oxygen transmissibility, but the diameter in and of itself is not responsible for the lens's advantages and disadvantages.

7. c) CAB is a gas permeable material. HEMA is the most common soft lens material. Sometimes other polymers are added to HEMA to enhance lens characteristics. Soft lenses also can be made of silicone polymers. Hydrogel is another word for soft lenses made of HEMA.

8. a) The lower the soft lens's water content, the more rigid it is, and hence, the more durable. Still, the soft lens does not approach rigidity in the sense that a hard or gas permeable lens does. A low water content lens is *less* oxygen transmissible.

9. b) As a rule, soft lenses (being soft and flexible) do not provide the crisp, sharp vision of rigid lenses.

10. a) If a hydrophilic lens doesn't get the water it "wants" from the tear film, its thickness (and thus, optics) can change. However, soft lenses correct spherical errors more successfully than astigmatic errors. An infant and a child are good candidates because the soft lens provides more comfort and a low rate of lens loss on impact. Rigid lenses may pop out on impact, which makes the soft lens a good choice for the recreational basketball player as well.

11. b) The soft lens's flexible nature also makes it vulnerable to problems of durability. The lens can be torn easily. (Nondisposable types may also crack or split with age. The life expectancy of a nondisposable soft lens is generally considered to be only about 1 year.) However, there is less lens loss, better oxygen permeability, and a low risk of injury on insertion (because the edges are soft).

12. c) The biggest risk listed is that of infection. The pores of soft lens material generally are too small for bacteria to penetrate. However, once the lens forms deposits, there is a rough surface on which bacteria may grow. In addition, the removal of a deposit may create a pit large enough to harbor bacteria. While it is true that modifications are impossible, residual astigmatism goes uncorrected, and the lenses can discolor, these hardly qualify as risks.

13. a) Lenticular astigmatism (astigmatism caused by irregular curvature of the crystalline lens, as opposed to the cornea) usually is corrected readily by soft toric lenses. Because lens stability is so important in toric lenses in order to keep the cylinder aligned, lid position and function are very important.

14. b) Keeping the cylinder properly aligned means keeping the lens aligned. A spherical lens normally is pushed around and rotated during blinking. This spells disaster for a toric lens fit.

15. Matching:
Aspheric back surface	e
Bioflange	f
Dynamic stabilization	c
Posterior toric	d
Prism ballast	a
Truncation	b

16. a) Double slab-off is another name for dynamic stabilization. The technique also is called "thick-thin zones" (see question 15, definition *c*).

17. b) Soft toric lenses have etch marks or dots either at the base or at the horizontal meridian. These can be observed with the slit lamp. The examiner looks for lens rotation as the patient blinks.

18. b) The acronym for compensating for axis misalignment is LARS: left, add, right, subtract. SAM (steeper add minus) FAP (flatter add plus) has to do with adjusting lens base curve and power. TAM is a friend of mine, and Roy G. Biv is an acronym to remember the colors of the spectrum.

19. d) The degrees of rotation are added to the patient's refraction.

20. b) Lens stability is influenced by the contour, position, and tightness of the lens. Weighting and truncation are the techniques used to cope with lens instability, but are not the cause of the instability. K readings are used to fit the lens, but are not the cause of instability. The thickness and water content are not factors either.

21. d) Rigid toric lenses might be the lens of choice when the K readings and refraction don't match either in power or in axis (answers *a* and *c*), as well as when there is lenticular astigmatism.

22. a) A rigid lens will rock on the steepest meridian. Vertical astigmatism may cause vertical decentration, and horizontal astigmatism may cause horizontal decentration. A larger lens may stabilize better.

23. b) Ultra-thin rigid lenses may flex on the eye, inducing astigmatism. Thus, a thicker or stiffer lens is required.

24. a) Astigmatism that is "left over" after the eye is fit with a contact lens is called *residual astigmatism*.

25. c) Residual astigmatism is most often caused by lenticular astigmatism, or irregular curvature of the crystalline lens (which doesn't show up on K readings).

26. c) A small amount of astigmatism in a spherical soft lens wearer is merely tolerated, not masked or eliminated. As long as the patient tolerates it, there is no reason to rush into fitting a toric lens.

27. a) As long as the astigmatism is less than 1/3 of the total refractive error, there is a good chance that the patient can tolerate the vision provided by a spherical soft contact lens.

28. d) If astigmatism is 3.00 diopters or less, it is generally adequate to fit a spherical rigid lens. The lens itself, by its position and tilt, may induce enough cylinder to compensate.

29. d) Simultaneous vision bifocal contacts are concentrically designed. The inner "bull's-eye" is for distance vision, and the outer ring is for near vision. Each eye is fit with such a lens. They are available in progressive style.

30. a) The size of the patient's pupil is a limiting factor in fitting concentric lenses. If the pupil is not large enough, the near vision may be restricted. If the pupil is too large, the patient may experience ghosting and flare from the transitions.

31. a) Ghost images are a frequent complaint. First, this is due to the transition area, or "line" between the segments. It is also due to the unfocused areas, or portions of what the patient is looking at (whether near or far) that fall into the "wrong" segment.

32. c) A reverse design simultaneous vision bifocal contact has the near portion in the center "bull's eye" and the distance portion in the outer ring. This takes advantage of the fact that pupil constriction is part of the accommodative reflex. When the patient views something up close, the pupils constrict, and the vision is "forced" through the central reading portion of the contact, eliminating ghosts from the outer distance portion.

33. b) The above effect can backfire, however. Pupil constriction also might be caused by bright light. The small pupil then restricts vision to the close-up central part of the lens. This is a major hazard if you are driving when it happens.

34. d) Alternating vision bifocal contact lenses are designed like bifocal glasses lenses. The upper portion is for distance and the lower segment is for near. Since people usually look down when holding reading material, this works well. Both eyes wear such a lens.

35. b) If the lower lid is at or just barely below the inferior limbus, the alternating vision bifocal contact will be in a good position. If the lid is abnormally high or low, the reading segment may not be in proper position for reading in down gaze.

36. b) Just like bifocal glasses, trying to see something close-up that is overhead is difficult because you are trying to read at mid-range through the distance segment. The object or print will be blurred.

37. c) The increased movement of the gas permeable lens makes it easier for the patient to "find" the right spot for close-up reading. The lens bumps into the lower lid margin, holding it steady as the pupil slides into down gaze for reading. A soft lens follows the eye's motion.

38. b) In the monovision technique, one eye (usually the dominant eye) is fitted for distance and the other eye is fitted for near. In some cases, the dominant eye might be fitted for near, but this is not the routine procedure.

39. c) Anyone who continuously works up close and requires "perfect" near vision all the time (such as a bookkeeper, accountant, etc) probably is not a good candidate for monovision. Monovision involves a trade-off. Both distance and near vision are somewhat compromised and binocular vision is sacrificed, but the patient doesn't have to cope with bifocals (glasses or contacts). Those people listed in the other answers do some up close work, but also need to look frequently at a distance to see their audience.

40. a) The test for the driver's exam is a distance vision test. Often the eye fit for near will fail to read the required distance figures. In this case, a letter or form may be required from the physician, explaining the situation.

41. d) The high success rate of IOLs has drastically reduced the need for fitting aphakes with contact lenses. While answers *b* and *c* are true, these reasons have not had a significant impact on the rate of aphakic fits.

42. b) The average aphakic may be an older patient, but certainly is not necessarily senile! However, older patients do tend to have dry eye, and have lost enough muscle tone that lid laxity can be a problem. Older patients also are more prone to superior corneal neovascularization because of the surgical wound as well as the heat that is generated under the upper lid, especially with a thick soft lens on the eye.

43. b) Images will appear to be smaller with high plus contacts than with high plus spectacles. Thus, the patient will have the impression that objects are farther away.

44. b) The aphakic patient cannot see up close without his glasses. Since glasses must be removed in order to insert contact lenses (soft or rigid), this is a problem. Several handy gadgets have been devised to assist high hyperopes with lens handling. Many aphakic patients can learn to handle the lenses, however, and a caregiver is not needed. An aphake does have corneal sensation. Soft lenses are not removed with a plunger.

45. c) A lenticular lens reduces the weight and mass of a high plus rigid lens. In addition, the thicker edges are "grabbed" by the upper lid, helping to pull up the lens and keep it in position.

46. a) The power of a high plus lenticular lens is ground on the bowl of the lens. (The other part of the lens, which provides the lens edges, is referred to as the *carrier*.)

47. d) A minus carrier is used for a high plus lens because it has a thin center and a thick edge. This is referred to as a *myoflange*. A *hyperflange* is a plus carrier. There is no such thing as a myoprism or a hyperprism.

48. c) See question 45.

49. b) A soft lens generally can be fit once there is no (absolutely *no*) corneal edema, often at 1 week postoperative.

50. a) If a soft lens is fit and worn in the presence of postoperative corneal edema, endothelial cells can be lost during a single day's wear.

51. d) A larger diameter soft lens will help stabilize the heavy high plus lens required for aphakia. Soft lenses are not fenestrated. A good aphakic fit with a soft lens will provide apical touch, vault the limbus, then make contact again at the lens periphery.

52. c) There is no connection between taking blood thinners and wearing contact lenses.

53. b) High water content extended wear soft lenses tend to develop deposits at an increased rate. A high water content lens does tend to move more than a low water content lens, but in dry eye there certainly would not be excess movement.

54. d) The reduced lens movement of the low water content extended wear soft lens means that it is more difficult for debris under the lenses to be flushed away. The lens, however, is more resistant to heat and deposits. High water content lenses tend to be sensitive to environmental changes. An arid or hot environment can cause the lenses to shrink and steepen, changing both the fit and the vision.

55. c) It is the current trend to advise that the patient remove extended wear lenses once a week, leaving them out overnight for cleaning. See question 54 for comments on low and high water content lenses. Neovascularization is more common in aphakes because of the surgical wound, lens thickness, and heat generated under the upper lid.

56. a) Every patient who wears contact lenses on an extended basis needs to lubricate the lenses regularly, especially every morning.

57. c) See question 56. It is not necessary for every patient to remove and clean the lenses every day, although some do and should. Nor is it advisable to blithely allow every patient to wear them for a month at a time. Most physicians recommend weekly removal. If the eye is red or painful, the lens must always be removed.

58. a) A gradual increase in myopia, seen in some extended wear patients, is caused by corneal edema. The edema can be so subtle that one might not be able to see it even with the slit lamp. If detected early and extended wear is discontinued, it probably will reverse itself.

59. b) It is generally recommended that extended wear soft contacts be replaced every 3 to 6 months, whether ruined by deposits or not.

60. a) Because of the oxygen transmissibility of the gas permeable material, neovascularization is less common than with soft lenses. While usually touted as not warping the cornea, distortion can occur in extended wear situations.

61. d) Studies show that an aphakic eye needs less oxygen (about 50% less) than a phakic eye.

62. b) Fit the loosest lens that will give good vision and comfort. Even if it looks like a "sloppy, floppy" fit, as long as the patient is comfortable and can see well, go with it.

63. a) Because a gas permeable lens allows more oxygen to get to the cornea, the eye can tolerate a larger lens. True, it is more comfortable than a PMMA lens, but this is due to the fit (sliding under the upper lid vs. bumping into it), not permeability. Lens movement still is important. The properly fit gas permeable lens does not sit on the lower lid.

64. c) The average life of a rigid gas permeable lens is 18 to 24 months. (The gas permeable material is not as tough as PMMA.)

65. d) The higher Dk value gas permeable lenses are more likely to warp. These lenses generally contain more silicone, making the lens a bit more flimsy. The items in the other answers are not factors.

66. b) An exophthalmic eye usually is fit better with a soft lens, which is more stable on the eye and doesn't interfere with the lids. Cases represented by the other answers are good candidates.

67. a) HEMA (hydroxyethyl methacrylate) is a soft lens material.

68. b) The more silicone content in a gas permeable lens, the higher the Dk value (oxygen transmission). Unfortunately, the high silicone content lenses tend to wet poorly, develop more deposits, and are less durable.

69. a) The upper lid should control the movement of the gas permeable lens. The lid should "grab" the lens, move it with each blink, and "hold" the lens up off the lower lid.

70. b) Gas permeable lenses develop fewer deposits than soft lenses, but they still develop deposits. Answers *a*, *c*, and *d* are true.

71. c) Truncation is removing a portion of the bottom of the lens to create a straight edge. This straight edge rides the lower lid margin and helps keep the soft toric lens from rotating, thus providing stability.

72. a) Truncation alone may not be enough to stabilize the lens, because the lens may rock back and forth (with accompanying changes in the cylinder axis, resulting in blurred vision). If a prism ballast is added, the flat lower portion of the lens is thicker and weighed down, reducing the seesaw motion.

73. d) Instead of dehydration and exposure of the superior cornea, it is the inferior cornea that can be dehydrated and exposed. Hence, the inferior staining and injection mentioned in answer *c* are possible problems. Difficulty with near vision comes when the patient looks down because the lower lid displaces the lens. Some patients complain of lens awareness as well, since the lens conforms to the lower lid margin.

74. b) Truncation is also used to stabilize bifocal contact lenses.

75. a) While a bandage lens of a specific power may be chosen, correcting the refractive error is not the priority in a bandage lens. In fact, a plano lens usually is preferred because it is thinner and thus more oxygen permeable.

76. c) Getting oxygen to the cornea is the key in selecting a bandage lens. A bandage lens generally is not handled by the patient. K readings may be taken and used, but not in every case.

77. b) See question 75.

78. c) A *high* water content lens is preferred because it is more oxygen permeable.

79. d) The routine no-stitch cataract surgery patient does not require a bandage lens as a regular procedure. In rare cases of wound leakage, a bandage lens might be used to help seal the wound and promote anterior chamber formation. A bandage lens is routine procedure following excimer laser surgery. Use of a bandage lens in corneal erosion or ulcer would be decided on a case-by-case basis.

80. a) The purpose of a drug reservoir is to absorb the drug and thus keep the external eye constantly exposed to the medication. A rigid lens can't do that. Answer *c* applies to the use of a lens as a splint, not as a drug reservoir. Not all soft lenses disintegrate, only the collagen lenses.

81. b) If the corneal surface is not intact, a tight-fitting lens is in order. If the corneal surface is intact, then you want 0.5 to 1.0 mm movement to allow for exchange of oxygen and waste products.

82. a) Discomfort may continue for a day or two in the case of a corneal abrasion or erosion, despite the presence of a bandage lens. The lens is not to be handled by the patient. Topical anesthetic is never prescribed for home use as it slows healing and compromises the corneal structure.

83. c) The Dk value is a laboratory measurement of the oxygen permeability of a material. The higher the Dk, the more permeable the material. That's not to say, however, that the Dk is a measurement of how much oxygen actually reaches the cornea (see question 84). True, the higher water content lenses are more permeable, but this is not the actual measurement of permeability. The wetting angle has to do with the degree to which a liquid (tears) "beads up" at the edge of the contact.

84. a) The oxygen that reaches the cornea is affected not only by the Dk value of the material, but by lens design (steep, flat, fenestrated, etc) and thickness (both of edges and periphery). An aphakic lens, for example, has a large central thickness and less oxygen transmissibility than a +3.00 lens. By contrast, a high minus lens is thicker at the periphery, which can also cut down on transmission of oxygen.

85. b) Oxygen circulates under a PMMA lens via the tears.

86. a) A high Dk value indicates greater oxygen permeability. A thinner lens also increases oxygen transmission to the cornea (see question 84).

87. a) If oxygen availability falls below 1.5 to 2.5%, corneal edema will result. The availability of oxygen in the atmosphere is 20%. During sleep (with no contact lens on the eye), the availability falls to about 7%.

88. d) The silicone lens has the highest Dk value of the lenses listed. PMMA is the plastic used in "old fashioned" hard lenses. HEMA is commonly used in soft lenses. CAB and silicon are gas permeable lens materials.

89. b) Radius is a line drawn from the center of a sphere to the edge. The base curve of a contact lens is actually the radius of the sphere to which the lens corresponds. Answer *a* describes circumference, and answer *c* defines diameter.

90. a) If the contact lens was a slice off of a sphere (which is equally curved in every direction), the sphere's radius would be the lens's base curve. A circle won't work because it's only two-dimensional; a sphere is three-dimensional. A cylinder and ellipse are not equally curved in all directions.

91. b) A longer radius corresponds to a flatter base curve. The longer the radius, the bigger the sphere from which the lens was "sliced." A slice of a big sphere would be flatter.

92. c) The vault of a lens describes the distance from the lens's center to a flat surface. A flatter lens would be closer to surface, thus it would have a lower vault. Base curve and radius are the same thing, and were defined above. Diameter is a measurement from one side of the lens to the other, running directly through the center of the lens.

93. a) This statement is the same as saying that the patient should be fit with the *tightest* lens possible. The opposite is true; the patient generally is fit with the loosest (lowest vault) possible. The other statements are true.

94. d) See question 92. (Sagittal depth is another term for vault.)

95. b) Increasing the lens' diameter increases vault and acts to tighten the lens.

96. c) Higher powered lenses are thicker, either in the center (plus lens) or at the edges (minus lens). Either way, this can create a decrease in the amount of oxygen getting to the cornea. Hypoxia is a lack of oxygen.

97. b) The higher the water content of a soft lens, the more oxygen can be transmitted to the cornea. Unfortunately, these lenses are sensitive to dehydration if the environment changes. They also are heat sensitive, and some types may not be disinfected using thermal methods. Given the same water content, the non-HEMA lenses are more durable.

98. a) The base curve of a rigid lens is on the central posterior curve. The intermediate and peripheral curves have a base curve of their own, but these are not considered the true base curve of the lens.

99. a) The optical zone of the lens is the portion that is intended to be positioned in front of the pupil. The lens power is ground on the optic zone. The junctions are the places where curves meet. There is no "limbal" zone. True, every curve has power, but the prescriptive power is on the optical zone.

100. d) The junctions between adjacent curves are blended, or smoothed, for comfort and centration. The blend might vary from light to heavy, and anywhere in between.

101. d) Beveling is used to taper the edges of a high minus rigid contact. (A minus lens is thinner in the middle and thicker at the edges.)

102. b) The tear film may create a "lens" (referred to as the *lacrimal lens*) under a rigid contact. If the contact is fit steeper than K, it will have a high vault. The tears under the contact will form a plus tear lens, and the contact will need to have minus power added to adjust. A lens fit flatter than K has a low vault, creating a minus tear lens. Plus power will need to be added to the contact to compensate. Axial length is not used in determining contact lens power, nor is a cell count. The size of the fovea is not a factor, either.

103. d) In addition to measuring the curvature of the central cornea, the keratometer can be used to identify warped and edematous corneas (the mires appear wavy, blurred, or discontinuous). A keratometer does not measure the corneal periphery (its main drawback), nor can one directly view a contact lens through it. Keratoconus is better evaluated via corneal topography.

104. Order:
    3 Occlude the eye not being tested
    5 Turn the drum so that the plus signs are aligned exactly tip-to-tip
    6 Turn the dials to superimpose the plus and minus signs
    2 Position the patient
    4 Focus the mires and center the cross-hairs in the lower right hand circle
    1 Focus the eyepiece
    Note: Steps 5 and 6 may be reversed, but most examiners prefer to set the axis before completing alignment.

105. c) The plus sign is projected on the side, and the main thing that might obstruct the mires from the side is the occluder on the keratometer. A common vertical obstruction (which would obstruct the *minus* signs) is the patient's upper lid.

106. Matching:
Flat cornea	d
Corneal warpage	f
Keratoconus	g
Spherical cornea	b
Steep cornea	a
Dry eye	e
Astigmatism	c

107. c) If the cross-hairs are not centered, you are not reading the corneal apex. Because the corneal periphery is flatter, the resulting fit will be too loose when placed on the steeper apex.

108. c) A soft lens fit steeper than K usually will have the effects of a steep lens: poor movement, a plus tear layer, fluctuations in vision when blinking, and discomfort. The vision usually is clearer right after the blink (when the apex of the lens is pushed onto the cornea) and blurs thereafter (when the apex of the lens pulls back off of the cornea).

109. a) See question 108.

110. c) Corneal edema causes steepening of the corneal curvature. Corneal molding, or warpage, generally causes flattening. Neovascularization has no direct effect on K readings. A corneal ulcer might cause distortion of the mires.

111. d) Any progressive change in the K readings of a contact lens wearer should be dealt with by changing lens material or design. Power changes might be required, but changing the power will not address the cause of the corneal change. Changing solutions would have no effect. The patient need not give up on contacts permanently at this point.

112. a) Fitting a lens "on K" means to match the base curve of the lens to the flattest corneal curve.

113. b) The methods in answers *a*, *b*, and *d* are all accurate. But for most purposes, measuring visible iris is good enough. A pachymeter measures corneal thickness.

114. a) The edges of a rigid lens should fall within the corneal diameter without limbal contact. A soft lens should overlap the limbus.

115. b) A patient with large pupils needs a larger optic zone and a larger lens for best vision. The risks and side effects associated with miotics make that option unacceptable.

116. d) If the pupil dilates beyond the optic zone, then light is coming through the peripheral curves into the eye. This causes glare and light flares. Answers *a* and *b* have to do with the steepness of the lens. A large pupil is not related to corneal edema.

117. a) If the tear BUT is 10 seconds or less, the tear film is considered subnormal.

118. a) A hydrophilic lens (hydro = water, philic = love) wants water. If it doesn't get it, it will pull any available fluid off the eye, drying a dry eye even more. In this situation, the lens has a tendency to get stuck, not move excessively.

119. d) As a soft lens dries out, its base curve (not diameter) changes, altering its optical qualities and producing blurred vision. Selected tear supplement drops can be used with soft lenses in place. The dry lens moves little if at all.

120. c) Excessive tears equal excessive movement as the lens floats around on the extra fluid. Answers *a*, *b*, and *d* are seen in a tight/dry lens situation.

121. d) A patient with dry eyes needs to take longer to build up rigid lens wearing time. The word "only" in answer *a* should have identified it as incorrect.

122. a) An interpalpebral lens fits within the lid fissures, so it is more likely to bump into the lids. There also is more opportunity for the lens to "center" with a peripheral curve in the patient's visual axis, causing glare and flare.

123. a) The lids are retracted in exophthalmos and unable to support a rigid lens properly. Lens support is not so critical in a soft lens fit.

124. c) An upper lid that grabs or pushes is a tight lid. A lax lid may move the lens little, if any.

125. Matching:

Horizontal band	f
Vertical band	g
3 and 9 o'clock staining	b
Diffuse staining	k
Dense apical staining	i
Diffuse apical staining	a
Zigzags	c
Arc stain	h
Pooling under lens center	e
Pooling under lens periphery	j
No stain under lens	l
No stain in intermediate zone	d

126. d) The closer you get to the retina, the more plus power it takes to converge and focus the image. So a hyperope may need more power in the contact than in the glasses. Aphakes also are hyperopes. A myope might need more plus, too (translating to *less* minus).

127. c) Compensate for vertex distance if the spherical power is 4.00 diopters or more. (Some references may say 3.00 diopters.)

128. b) Minus cylinder form is used for rigid lens power calculation. Spherical equivalent is used in soft lenses. See question 127 about vertex distance.

129. b) When fitting a low power spherical rigid lens on K, just use the spherical portion of the refractometric measurement. No other calculating is needed.

130. a) When fitting on K (42.0), select a power of -2.50. But you are fitting 0.50 diopters steeper than K. In order to go steeper, it is necessary to add minus to compensate, diopter for diopter. So add -0.50 to -2.50 = -3.00. (Remember SAM? Steeper Add Minus.)

131. c) The power of a soft spherical contact is chosen by the spherical equivalent of the refractometric measurement. The K readings are not used for calculating the power.

132. d) To find the spherical equivalent, add half of the cylinder to the sphere, then drop the cylinder and axis.

133. d) The spherical equivalent is necessary since you are fitting a soft spherical contact. Half of the cylinder is +0.50. Add this to the sphere power: -3.00 + 0.50 = -2.50.

134. d) When fitting a soft toric, you want the least amount of cylinder correction that the patient will accept, because the lens will rotate a bit on the eye. The higher the amount of cylinder, the more pronounced the visual problems caused by this rotation.

135. a) Over-refractometry is used to refine the power of the contact lens, and has little application in answers *b* through *d*.

136. c) You always want to encourage the patient to take as much plus as possible to prevent accommodation. Translated, this means giving the most plus (or subtracting the least).

137. a) If the patient is presbyopic, find out how the lenses are fit before pulling the refractor forward. Are they monofit? Bifocals? Maybe distance OU with reading glasses? Knowing what to expect before you start will make your job easier.

138. c) Residual astigmatism (the amount of astigmatism that is not corrected by the contact lens) is usually due to lenticular astigmatism, or irregular curvature of the crystalline lens inside the eye.

139. d) You can generally ignore residual astigmatism of 0.50 or less when fitting a soft spherical contact.

140. d) The lenses are switched. The over-refractometry is of equal amounts but opposite signs, which is the big giveaway. The least myopic eye, now wearing a stronger lens, can accommodate and still see 20/20. The more myopic eye, now wearing a weaker lens, simply cannot see as well.

141. c) Leave her lenses on and look at her with the slit lamp. Chances are the lenses are coated with hair spray or something similar. But if the contacts look clear, remove them and check for corneal haze. Another option is to do a pin hole vision. If it helps, possibly check to see if the lenses in the refractor are clean. If it doesn't help, you're back to using the slit lamp. If the lenses are crossed, you should be able to clear the vision with refractometry as above.

142. a) Unilateral aphakia creates anisometropia, which, in the pediatric patient, leads to amblyopia. The aphakic eye must be corrected with a contact, since glasses would not be tolerated (due to the big difference between the refractive error of the eyes).

143. c) If the pediatric contact lens fit is to be successful, the parent must be highly motivated.

144. b) The silicone lens is the lens of choice to correct aphakia in children. Soft lenses usually are not available in the small diameter required. The "breathability" of silicone surpasses that of other lens materials.

145. d) If selecting a soft lens for a small child or infant, you need to know if the lens can be designed with a steep enough base curve, small enough diameter, and high enough power. The optic zone varies with diameter. If anything, you would want a larger optic zone to account for the large pupils found in children.

146. a) An aphakic infant is usually fit to focus on close objects, because a baby's world mostly exists within his own reach. An aphake cannot accommodate, ruling out answer c. Fitting on the minus side would extend the focus beyond near range.

147. a) Toric lenses are not fit on infants as a general rule. Options b through d are viable, although d is not ideal.

148. b) A soft extended wear lens will relieve the parents from having to handle the lenses every day. However, these lenses are more flimsy (and hence less durable), tend to fold up when handled, and are more easily rubbed out of the eye and lost.

149. b) A child should be taught how to remove and insert the lenses as soon as she is old enough to do so.

150. c) A patient who works around smoke, dust, and fumes still can wear contacts, just not at work!

151. a) Contact sports often involve blows to the head, which might pop out a rigid lens. Presbyopes can wear soft or rigid lenses. A person with very mild dexterity problems probably can handle a rigid lens *more* easily. Rigid lenses generally give sharper, more stable vision, and would be ideal for a compulsive person.

152. b) Many practitioners agree that a person who wants contacts only for cosmetic reasons, and doesn't need them for improved vision, is taking more risk than the benefit is worth. The 50-year-old may be emmetropic, but she also is presbyopic, and may warrant a contact lens in one eye for near, or a set of bifocal contacts. The teen and aphake probably will be very motivated.

153. b) A history of episcleritis does not make one a poor contact lens candidate. The patient with the pinguecula might get by with an intrapalpebral fit. The pterygium creates an irregular corneal surface. The patient in answer a is the poorest candidate of all.

154. d) Propine is an epinephrine derivative that can discolor soft lenses. She should be fit with rigid lenses.

155. b) The patient who has had glaucoma filtration surgery has a drainage blister, or bleb, between the sclera and conjunctiva. The bleb would interfere with the way the lens rides on the eye. All the other patients can be fit.

156. b) Diabetes is not necessarily associated with dry eye.

157. a) Patients should be given a training session that includes verbal instruction, plus written instructions to refer to at home. Providing only written instruction or no written material at all is an invitation to failure. Trusting patient instruction to other patients (who may or may not remember *their* instructions) is ill-advised.

158. c) Patients should be taught to wash their hands before handling lenses. This is one of the rare times where "always" does not signal a wrong answer! Its use in answer a renders it incorrect, however.

159. a) Patients can be taught to recognize an inverted lens by both visual inspection and the taco test. There's no such thing as the jelly roll test or an inversion tester.

160. c) Inserting a soft lens is easiest if the lens is wet (not dripping) and the finger is dry (to prevent sticking).

161. a) The nondominant hand is used to pin the upper lid to the brow to prevent blinking. The lens itself is best handled with the dominant hand.

162. a) The lens should be placed directly on the cornea, bull's-eye style. Sliding isn't a good idea with a rigid lens, as this can cause a corneal abrasion. A lens on the lid margin is almost sure to be blinked out.

163. d) Soft lenses are pinched out with thumb and forefinger at the 9 and 3 o'clock positions. A plunger could tear a soft lens. Blinking and squeezing don't work.

164. c) Long fingernails are the nemesis of soft contact lenses. A person who is unwilling to cut the nails can learn to adapt, however, by turning the fingers to keep the nails away from the lens and eye.

165. b) Blinking out a rigid lens requires the patient to look down, open both eyes wide, and pull the temporal canthus with thumb or finger. The lens must be centered on the eye for this to work.

166. c) Teach your patients never to apply the plunger to the eye unless they know exactly where the contact lens is. "Fishing" for a lost lens with the plunger is disastrous, and painful if the plunger adheres to cornea or sclera. A drop of wetting solution helps the lens stick to the plunger, and carrying an extra plunger is always a good idea.

167. a) Body temperature grunge is easier to remove. A soft lens should not be allowed to dry out.

168. b) Neither cleaning nor disinfecting is optional. Disinfectant can't reach all the surfaces of a dirty lens. Cleaning removes dirt, film, and deposits; disinfectant kills germs.

169. b) The lens should be cleaned gently by a fingertip as the lens rests on the palm. The pressure between the thumb and forefinger is too great. In order for the cleaner to be effective, there must be some physical friction; little, if any, cleaning takes place when the cleaner is applied and rinsed off without any rubbing.

170. a) A rigid lens that is stored dry for a period of time can warp.

171. c) If a gas permeable lens dries out, the base curve may change. It should return to normal after soaking for 4 hours or overnight.

172. d) In order for disinfection to be maintained, the disinfecting solution should be changed daily. Adding a little active disinfectant to a chamber of old disinfectant dilutes the active solution, rendering it too weak for the purpose. Saline (preserved or otherwise) does not disinfect.

173. a) To prevent a filmy build-up on the lens, only hand soap that is free of moisturizers and other additives should be used. Make up, face cream, and hair spray should be used before inserting lenses. Hand lotion should be used after.

174. c) A dropped lens should be cleaned and disinfected before wearing. No exceptions.

175. b) The contact lens case should *not* be washed with soap because residue could interfere with the disinfectant or cause a film on the lenses. The entire case should be replaced every couple of months.

176. b) Wetting solutions, used with rigid lenses, are used to cause the tear film to spread evenly over the lens. This increases comfort. Wetting solution does not sterilize, reduce deposits, or prevent scratches.

177. a) Gross as it may be, urine is more sterile than saliva. (Telling your patients this may discourage the terrible habit of wetting a rigid lens in the mouth!) Saliva harbors all kinds of nasty, infection-causing bacteria. Tap water and pool water (although "cleaner" than saliva) are not the right solutions, either, and can cause the lens to adhere to the cornea, as well as corneal edema.

178. a) The surfactant acts to clean the surface of the lens. It is not used to soak or rewet. It is toxic to the eye and should never be instilled directly into the eye.

179. c) Enzyme cleaners are used to remove protein build-up on soft and gas permeable lenses. They do not provide the advantages listed in answers a, b, or d.

180. c) *Acanthamoeba* has been linked with homemade saline from salt tablets and distilled water.

181. a) The combination soak and wet solutions do not eliminate the all-important first step of surface cleaning.

182. d) Patients should understand that contact lens solutions are chemicals that do not always mix well with each other. Although they need not buy only from your office, they should use one solution system and stick with it unless problems develop.

183. a) A rigid lens has a longer wearing time building schedule than a soft lens (answers b through d).

184. c) The upper limit recommended for daily contact lens wear is 15 hours a day.

185. c) Contact lens fitters vary in their recommended wearing schedule. Among the answers offered, wear three, remove one, wear three is the best selection.

186. b) Once a rigid lens wearer has worked up to 5 or 6 hours a day, an additional hour of wear can be added every other day.

187. b) Full wearing time for a rigid lens wearer can be achieved (in the absence of problems) in 4 to 5 weeks.

188. b) Soft lenses may be worn 8 to 10 hours on the first day.

189. a) It takes about a week (barring problems) for a soft lens wearer to build up to full-time daily wear.

190. c) Symptoms usually start 2 to 3 hours after removing the lenses.

191. a) The typical slit lamp findings in OWS are diffuse apical erosions that stain deeply with fluorescein.

192. d) Before the new contact lens wearer walks out the door, the final, cardinal rule to be emphasized is to remove a lens if the eye becomes red and/or painful. No exceptions.

193. a) Problems associated with a tight lens include corneal edema, sensations of soreness, injection, foggy vision, and ghost images. Answers b and d go with a loose lens. Allergies to solutions don't affect the fit per se.

194. c) Edge standoff is a sign of a loose lens.

195. c) A tight lens is a steep lens. When the patient blinks, the apex of the contact is pushed onto the apex of the cornea, clearing the vision. After a second or two, the lens pops back off the cornea and the vision blurs. The opposite is true of a loose, flat lens.

196. a) A tight lens can be loosened by decreasing the diameter or flattening the base curve. Either one of these solutions makes the lens flatter and looser. Doing the opposite would make the lens even tighter, as would increasing the vault. Vertex distance has nothing to do with the lens' physical fit.

197. b) A loose lens is a flat lens. There is often edge standoff, which can cause a foreign body sensation. A loose lens also exhibits excessive movement. If the lens slips off center when the patient moves his eyes, vision will blur. Power and hygiene do not come into play.

198. d) As mentioned above, a loose lens will move excessively and tend to slip off center. The standoff edges may tend to pucker as they are pushed around by the eyelids.

199. b) A loose lens may be tightened by increasing lens diameter or steepening the base curve. Either of these measures will cause the curve of the lens to conform more to the curve of the eye. (A thinner lens also may work because it will adhere to the cornea better.)

200. a) Vascularization, or the development of new, abnormal blood vessels in the cornea, results from a lack of oxygen (hypoxia).

201. b) The superior limbal area of the cornea (under the upper lid) is most often the spot where vascularization occurs.

202. d) An aphake who is wearing extended wear soft lenses is more at risk for developing vascularization than any other situation listed. Vascularization occurs more often with extended wear soft lenses to begin with. The aphakic cornea has also been traumatized by surgery.

203. b) Changing solutions won't affect neovascularization, which is not an allergic response to begin with. A looser, thinner, or higher water content lens would allow more oxygen to get through.

204. d) A rigid lens that does not center properly and continually rubs on the limbus may stimulate the growth of corneal blood vessels. It should ride on the central cornea, be lifted, and then drop a bit with each blink. Enzymatic cleaner will have little effect, if any.

205. b) *Pseudomonas* ulcers are more common in extended wear soft lenses. The sleeping eye is the type of warm, oxygen-poor environment in which bacteria thrive.

206. a) A corneal ulcer is not caused by sensitivity to contact lens chemicals. It is possible for a chemical keratitis to develop if solutions not meant for use directly in the eye are instilled by mistake, but that is different from an ulcer. Corneal ulcers associated with contact lens wear may be due to infection, trauma, or lack of oxygen.

207. d) Although gas permeable contact lens wearers may develop ulcers, they usually are not related to the lens itself. Ulcers are more commonly seen with soft contact lens wear.

208. b) Spectacle blur is the phenomenon noticed by contact lens wearers when they remove their contacts and experience blurred vision with their glasses. This blur can last from several minutes to weeks.

209. d) Spectacle blur is due to corneal edema (excess fluid in the cornea because of hypoxia) and/or corneal molding (where the cornea's shape is altered by the pressure of the contact lens).

210. a) Spectacle blur has long been associated with PMMA contact lens wearers, to the point where the phrase "contact lens addict" was coined. Contact lens addicts are PMMA wearers who increase their wearing time because of spectacle blur, unaware that by doing so they are making the situation worse.

211. b) Gas permeable contact lenses reduce the amount of noticeable spectacle blur. While corneal edema may occur with gas permeable contact lenses, the edema is more diffuse (spread evenly over the corneal surface), instead of central as with PMMA lenses.

212. a) GPC is considered to be an allergic response of the body to the protein deposits on a contact lens (usually soft). As the deposits break down, an allergic response is triggered.

213. c) The signs and symptoms of GPC include itching, mucus, lens intolerance, and the formation of large papillae on the inner surface of the upper eyelid. (The palpebral conjunctiva lines the lids; the bulbar conjunctiva covers the sclera.)

214. b) Because a larger lens means increased contact with the palpebral conjunctiva, it is felt that a lens over 14.0 mm in diameter can aggravate GPC.

215. d) See question 212.

216. c) New lenses with an admonition to keep them meticulously clean are in order. Heat disinfection is used rarely these days. Extended wear lenses are more likely to be associated with GPC problems due to increased opportunity for protein build-up and lens contact with the upper lid. Vasoconstrictor drops may decrease the redness, but will not address the allergic component of the problem.

217. a) A foreign body sensation is the most common symptom of lens deposits. The deposits rub on the cornea, creating discomfort and perhaps corneal abrasions.

218. c) "Jelly bumps" form when calcium and lipids (fat or oil) precipitate out of the tear film and onto the lens.

219. a) The silicone lens attracts lipids (fats and oils), so it tends to form a waxy coating. Jelly bumps are indigenous to soft lenses.

220. b) As a lens becomes coated with deposits, its ability to transmit oxygen decreases.

221. b) Protein deposits leave a pit in the lens when removed. Answers *a*, *c*, and *d* are all true. Enzyme cleaner acts on protein and other deposits by "digesting" them.

222. b) A lens with protein deposits is an ideal place for bacteria to grow. The eye is warm and moist, and the protein is food.

223. Matching/label:

A. Vascularization	b) no physical symptoms
B. Adaptation to new lenses	a) discomfort is a common complaint at first
C. Lens switch	b) causes a change in vision, not physical comfort
D. Foreign body	a)
E. Inverted lens	a) creates edge standoff and thus lens awareness
F. Vertex distance not accounted for	b)
G. Corneal abrasion	a)
H. Incorrect power	b) no physical symptoms
I. GPC	a) papillae on lid rub over eye, causing foreign body sensation
J. Lens overwear	a) moderate to severe pain starts several hours after lenses are removed
K. Corneal edema	b) painless
L. Infection	a)
M. Lens deposits	a) rub over the cornea
N. Tight lens	a) or b) may cause a sensation of soreness; many times, however, there is no discomfort
O. Loose lens	a) edge stand-off and excess movement = discomfort
P. Change in prescription	b)
Q. Toxic reaction to solutions	a) can cause painful chemical burn
R. Corneal ulcer	a)
S. Torn lens	a) torn edge rubs on the limbus, causing discomfort
T. Rigid lens crazing	b) these are not chips or deposits, and cause no physical discomfort
U. Smooth lens edges	b) *rough* edges cause discomfort

V. Fenestrated lens
W. Limbal touch

X. Excessive movement

b)
a) a rigid lens should ride within limbal boundaries, and a soft lens should cover over the limbus. The limbus has more sensation than the cornea, so limbal rub can be uncomfortable.
a) uncomfortable in both soft and rigid lenses

224. d) A well-fit rigid lens may not be a well-finished lens. If you cannot do the blending and polishing yourself, send the lens back to the lab.

225. c) The hypoxia associated with PMMA lenses causes a loss of corneal sensitivity as the nerve endings necrose (die). This is reversed when gas permeable materials are used. Corneal sensitivity recovers as the nerve endings regenerate, so the patient begins to feel the lenses. This actually is a good sign, which will decrease again as the patient adapts.

226. b) A corneal topography shows the curvature of the entire cornea. The keratometer only measures the corneal apex, which is only moderately useful. Placido's disk gives a picture of the curves, but no measurements. Pachymetry measures corneal thickness.

227. a) In the early stages, the keratoconus patient may be successfully corrected with soft lenses (spherical or toric) and glasses. Less is better, so save the rigid and specialty lenses until they are needed.

228. b) Mild keratoconus can be fit with gas permeable lenses. (See question 227.)

229. b) As the cone steepens, a rigid lens is needed in order to provide a smooth refractive surface. Since the contact is manufactured, it is a "perfect" surface used to cover the "imperfect" cone. In the effort to obtain good vision in keratoconus, getting rid of glasses is not the issue.

230. d) A smaller rigid lens is required to avoid the steeper peripheral curves. Totally vaulting the apex is not necessary. A bit of apical touch is allowable as long as the lens moves well enough to allow good tear exchange. Limbal touch is not desirable (and probably not possible).

231. c) The specialty lenses listed are designed to vault the corneal apex while still providing good movement.

232. b) Corneal edema is caused by a lack of oxygen to the cornea.

233. d) Symptoms of corneal edema include blurred vision, halos around lights, redness, and burning.

234. b) If a patient wearing extended wear contact lenses develops edema, try refitting with a different material or water content. A larger lens or increased wearing time will tend to make the problem worse. You probably fit the lens on K to begin with.

235. d) A rigid lens wearer who develops edema needs to have increased tear exchange under the lens, which will increase the oxygen available to the cornea. Choices *a* through *c* would *decrease* the tear exchange.

236. c) Statements *a*, *b*, and *d* are false. *Pseudomonas aeruginosa* and *Acanthamoeba* keratitis have been associated strongly with those who make their own saline from salt tablets.

237. d) Some preservatives and chemicals are not compatible, and may even set up an undesirable chemical reaction. Contamination is not the issue here, although if an old bottle of solution is contaminated and mixed with new solution, the new bottle becomes contaminated as well.

238. c) Thimerosal sensitivity is the most common chemical sensitivity problem with contact and other eye solutions. With so many nonpreserved solutions available, thimerosal reactions are becoming a thing of the past. Failing to disinfect after enzymatic cleaning causes problems, but is not as common as thimerosal. Chlorhexidine does not cause a reaction in and of itself, but rather causes uncomfortable dry spots on the lens. *Acanthamoeba* is out there, but is not common.

239. c) Switching to nonpreserved solutions and hydrogen peroxide-based cold disinfection often resolves the problem. There is no need to give up lenses without trying this first. Cleaning and storing lenses in unpreserved saline does not get the lenses clean nor does it disinfect, and therefore is not a good practice. Having the patient try various solutions on his own is not a good idea (see question 237).

240. d) An aphakic lens is a "huge" plus lens, thick in the center and thin on the edges. The myoflange increases edge thickness to provide for better lens movement.

241. a) Of the modifications listed, it is impossible to increase the diameter of a rigid lens by modification. You can reduce what is already there, but you cannot add what already has been taken away.

242. c) It is possible to reduce the power (ie, add minus) of a rigid lens by intense polishing, but only by about 0.50 diopters. The situations in answers *a*, *b*, and *d* all need more plus.

243. b) Remember the mnemonic SAM/FAP: steeper add minus, flatter add plus.

244. b) Fenestration indirectly increases oxygen to the cornea by improving tear exchange. The hole equalizes the pressure on both sides of the lens. The goal is not better movement in and of itself. Discomfort is not an indication to fenestrate, except that it can be caused by lack of oxygen.

245. c) Hypoxia (lack of oxygen) takes a few hours to build up before visual symptoms are noticed.

246. b) Vision that fluctuates with blinking is often associated with a loose or tight lens (see question 195). The word "always" in answer *d* should have been a red flag that it is incorrect.

247. b) A tight or loose lens is not the only thing that can cause vision to fluctuate with a blink. If there is excessive movement, the patient may not be looking through the optic zone. Vision through a peripheral part of the lens will not be as sharp. Fitting a lens with a larger optic zone might be part of the answer, along with reducing the movement.

248. b) Blurring after reading for long periods of time is usually due to dehydration. The patient gets so intent on reading that she forgets to blink. The same thing can happen when watching TV or working on a computer. You weren't given enough information (ie, the patient's age) to decide if the patient was presbyopic or not.

249. d) See answer 248. If the lens and cornea look good, try having the patient use rewetting drops before you go into a lot of fitting changes. The other items can cause blurring, but dehydration is the most common.

250. b) Any time a contact lens wearer is having a vision problem, the prime task is to determine whether it is in the contact lens or the cornea. Once you know which, then you can determine a course of action. The other items are important, but answer *b* is paramount.

251. a) In high power plus lenses, the power will differ depending on which way the lens is read. This is important when ordering and verifying high plus lenses. See question 252.

252. b) To read the back vertex power of a rigid contact, place the concave surface toward the lens stop. To read front vertex power, place the convex surface toward the lens stop.

253. d) The truncation or markings of a toric lens must be aligned to the bottom of the lens when placed into the lensometer. This simulates proper placement on the eye where the truncation or mark rides at 6:00.

254. c) Toric lens power and axis can be measured with a Tori-check device. The lens is put into the Tori-check and the device is placed onto the lensometer. Alignment is checked at the slit lamp with the lens on the eye. "Toric lens balance" is something I made up.

255. c) A soft contact lens can be read on the lensometer if it is gently blotted with a lint-free tissue and read quickly before it dehydrates. It can be read using a wet cell, but that is not the *only* way to read the lens.

256. b) The radiuscope is used to measure the base curve of rigid lenses, as well as to provide information about the lens surface.

257. c) The contact is placed concave side up when being read on the radiuscope.

258. Order:
    5 Focus the spoke image and set the measuring scale to zero
    6 Raise the microscope until the aerial image is seen
    2 Raise the microscope and focus the measuring scale
    7 Take the reading
    3 Lower the microscope until the lamp filament image is seen
    1 Center the contact and lens mount
    4 Lower the microscope further until the spoke target is seen

259. b) In some cases, the measuring scale may not set to zero. In this situation, set the scale to the nearest whole number. If you select +1.00, as in the test question, you will need to add 1.00 mm to the final reading. If you set the scale in the main part of the measuring scale, you will need to subtract that number from the final reading.

260. d) Keratometry and refractometry indicate that the patient does not have an appreciable amount of astigmatism, so the patient would not have been fit with a toric lens. This lens is warped. If a lens is toric or warped, all of the spoke lines will not be clear at the same time.

261. d) To evaluate for warpage, one should look at the aerial mires.

262. c) The base curve of a soft lens can be evaluated by placing the lens on a plastic template. If there is a bubble under the lens, then the lens is steeper than the template. If the edges of the lens stand off the template, then the lens is flatter than the template.

263. c) A rigid lens should be allowed to roll gently into place in the V-groove. It should not be pushed or forced. The lens need not be wet.

264. d) To read the lens diameter on the V-groove, read the scale mark nearest the center of the lens.

265. b) The diameter of a soft lens can be measured on a magnified see-through scale. The lens should not be smashed flat. Lens diameter of hydrogel lenses can be measured on a Soft Lens Analyzer, but that is not the *only* way to do it.

266. c) A central thickness gauge is used on rigid lenses. It would indent a soft lens.

267. d) The thickness gauge must be set to zero before using. (There is no eyepiece.)

268. a) A microscope or magnifier can be used to evaluate the edges of a soft contact lens. The Soft Lens Analyzer is designed for use on hydrogel lenses, not other kinds. A profile analyzer is used on rigid lenses. The lensometer is used to read lens power.

269. b) A profile analyzer is used to evaluate the curves of rigid lenses. There is no such thing as an edging gauge.

270. c) A well-blended rigid lens will have smooth, curving "ski" contours.

Chapter 6. Intermediate Tonometry

1. b) The ciliary body, at the base of the iris (but not the iris itself), is responsible for aqueous production.

2. a) Blood plasma is most like aqueous in composition, with some difference in trace elements.

3. d) The aqueous flows out of the posterior chamber, through the pupil into the anterior chamber, and then through the angle.

4. b) The flow of aqueous humor exiting the angle goes through the trabecular meshwork, into the canal of Schlemm, and from there into the episcleral veins. (Remember that veins carry blood to the heart. Arteries bring blood to an organ.)

5. b) IOP results from the combination of the amount of aqueous produced over time and its ability to drain out of the eye.

6. d) In order to lower the IOP (theoretically, at least), decrease the amount of aqueous being produced and/or increase the draining of it.

7. c) While slight, the aqueous *does* exert a refractive influence on light entering the eye. Response *a* refers to the diurnal curve of intraocular pressure, where IOP tends to be higher in the morning than in the evening. (In monitoring glaucoma, many physicians will vary the time of day that a patient comes in for IOP checks, to get a more clear idea of how treatment is affecting the pressure.) The IOP is slightly higher in the posterior chamber because the aqueous meets some resistance as it encounters the margin of the pupil. The circulating aqueous also acts to bring nutrients to and remove wastes from the eye's internal structures.

8. a) There is no indication that a patient with hypertension is at a higher risk of developing glaucoma. Answers *b* through *d do* indicate an increased risk. FYI: A recent study[1] indicates that patients with a central corneal thickness of 555 μm or less had a 3X *greater* chance of developing open-angle glaucoma. Whether the presence of diabetes increases the risk of glaucoma is under debate.

9. c) The fact that glaucoma screening generates public interest is not a plague, but a benefit. The other answers are problems inherent to screening programs.

10. c) Open-angle glaucoma is the most common type of glaucoma. (According to one source, there are over 40 different types of glaucoma.)

11. d) The classic hallmarks of glaucoma are increased IOP, loss of peripheral vision, and damage to the optic nerve head.

12. c) Retinoscopy is used to evaluate refractive errors, not glaucoma.

13. a) Gonioscopy uses a goniolens (a contact lens utilizing several mirrors) and a slit lamp to view the angle structures.

14. d) Unfortunately, vision lost due to glaucoma is not recoverable even once the condition is controlled or treated.

15. b) The diurnal curve of the IOP in a patient with glaucoma may vary up to 10 mm, being higher in the morning. The average (nonglaucomatous) eye varies only by about 4 mm. Thus, this larger fluctuation is a factor in both diagnosis and treatment of glaucoma. See also question 7.

16. d) An attack of angle-closure glaucoma can include signs and symptoms as follows: redness, hazy cornea, mid-dilated pupil (not miotic), pain, vomiting, nausea, headache, eye ache, halos around lights, and decreased vision.

17. c) A subconjunctival hemorrhage is red, but not painful.

18. a) When angle-closure glaucoma occurs, the iris is pushing against the lens and angle. Aqueous production continues, but the fluid is not drained out, causing a rise in IOP. If the pupil were miotic, as suggested in answer c, the iris would be pulled *away* from the angle, increasing drainage.

19. a) The pupil in angle-closure glaucoma is mid-dilated. Miotics are used in an effort to constrict the pupil and pull the iris out of the angle. Mydriatics would keep the pupil dilated. Antibiotics would have no effect, nor would corticosteroids. (Steroids can elevate the pressure when used for a period of time.)

20. c) Answers a, b, and d all act to dilate the pupil, creating a potential for the iris to block the angle. A sudden bright light would cause the pupil to constrict.

21. a) The eye of a high hyperope is short, meaning there is not much room for the angle. This increases the chances of iris obstruction. It is also the reason that we check angle depth prior to dilation, to make sure the angle is not going to occlude during mydriasis or cycloplegia.

22. b) Corneal edema has a prismatic effect, breaking light into its component colors, and thus creating halos around lights. Pressure build-up during an attack causes a breakdown in the pumping function of the corneal endothelium, and edema results.

23. b) Open-angle glaucoma cannot be cured; it can only be controlled. (In this respect, it resembles diabetes and high blood pressure.) Answers a, c, and d are true.

24. c) Because open-angle glaucoma has no physical symptoms, the patient is not driven to seek attention. The loss of peripheral vision occurs over a long period of time, often escaping the patient's notice. (Signs are perceptible to the examiner, such as optic disc cupping or an elevated IOP reading.)

25. d) As its name implies, the angle structure in open-angle glaucoma is open. Generally, it looks normal.

26. d) A patient with open-angle glaucoma needs an annual full exam including dilation, gonioscopy, and formal visual fields testing. Of course, he also needs periodic IOP checks during the year. The air-puff tonometer is not accurate enough to monitor glaucoma. Likewise, confrontation fields are not sensitive enough to monitor for field loss in glaucoma. Generally, it is safe to dilate a patient with open-angle glaucoma.

27. a) In advanced open-angle glaucoma, often the patient retains a small temporal island of vision. Eventually that is lost as well.

28. d) A patient with glaucoma who misses a pressure check undoubtedly should be contacted to reschedule. The importance of the exam and the gravity of the disease should be stated. Answers a and c border on neglect. Answer b is a breach of patient confidentiality.

29. b) There normally is a small depression, known as the physiologic cup, where the optic nerve enters the eye through the sclera, and through which the optic fibers pass.

30. c) In glaucoma, the pressure is transferred to the back of the eye where it can "excavate" the optic nerve. This causes the cup to be enlarged and caved-in, known as *cupping*. The blood vessels may dip over the cup's edge, but this in itself is not referred to as cupping.

31. b) The cup-to-disc ratio compares the amount of normal tissue to diseased tissue in the optic nerve head.

32. b) A large cup would be 0.9. In this case, 90% of the disc has been cupped out.

33. d) The normal disc is slightly oval in the horizontal direction. A cup that is vertical is very suspicious of glaucoma.

34. a) Because of the pattern of nerve fibers, optic nerve fiber damage is correlated to specific patterns of loss on the visual field. *Note:* See Chapter 7 for more on glaucoma medications.

35. d) Patient education is the key to successful treatment of glaucoma using medications. The patient should be told to continue the medication (including refilling it *before* it runs out) until instructed otherwise. In addition, the medication should be used on schedule, even (especially) when the patient has an appointment that day; otherwise it is more difficult to assess the treatment's efficacy.

36. c) If the patient understands the gravity of the disease, he will be *more* motivated to use the medication. Answers *a*, *b*, and *d* are common reasons for noncompliance.

37. b) Topical medications are usually the treatment of choice in open-angle glaucoma.

38. b) Steroids have the potential to raise the IOP in sensitive individuals if used over a period of time. Drugs in categories *a*, *c*, and *d* are used to treat glaucoma. Other categories of glaucoma medications are miotics and alpha-2 agonists.

39. a) Since miotics make the pupil smaller, a person with a subcapsular cataract (which occurs in the center of the lens) would experience more problems with decreased vision than the situations mentioned in answers *b* through *d*. Peripheral cortical cataracts occur in the outside edge of the lens, and probably would interfere very little, if any, once the pupil was constricted. Miotics also can cause accommodative spasms. However, aphakes and individuals over 65 have little or no accommodative abilities and would not notice these visual changes.

40. c) Of the drug types listed, most physicians prefer to use beta blockers as a first choice when instituting glaucoma therapy. Epinephrine derivatives and miotics are gradually fading from common use. Osmotics generally are used in angle-closure glaucoma.

41. b) As a group, beta blockers can interfere with respiratory function and are not given to patients with asthma or other lung conditions. *Note:* Certain beta blockers are less likely to have this side effect, however, and are sometimes prescribed.

42. b) Oral glycerin is a sickly-sweet liquid, so it usually is mixed with juice and poured over ice. The patient should sip it slowly.

43. a) A laser trabeculoplasty, the current most popular laser treatment for open-angle glaucoma, is directed at the trabecular meshwork in an attempt to increase aqueous drainage.

44. a) A laser iridotomy is used to create an opening in the iris to prevent pressure build-up in angle-closure glaucoma. Answers *b* and *c* require conventional surgery. Answer *d* refers to destruction of the iris, which is not done.

45. c) In procedures to treat angle-closure glaucoma, the idea is to allow the aqueous to flow between the anterior and posterior chambers.

46. c) Laser treatment can be accompanied by a rise (usually temporary) in the IOP.

47. a) A trabeculectomy is the name of the surgical procedure for glaucoma where a new drainage channel is created from the anterior chamber to the outside.

48. b) In a trabeculectomy, the aqueous is drained to an area under the conjunctiva. This creates a little sac or bleb.

49. c) The most common reason for bleb failure is a build-up of scar tissue. (Cystic fibrosis is a respiratory disease.)

50. a) Since the ciliary body produces the aqueous, some surgical procedures are aimed at destroying all or a part of the ciliary body in order to reduce the amount of aqueous being secreted into the eye.

    Note: As of publication, the topic of indentation tonometry has been moved from the COA® to the COT exam.

51. d) Indentation tonometry, as its name implies, measures how much the cornea can be indented by a given weight. (Applanation tonometry measures how much force it takes to flatten a specific area of cornea.)

52. b) When the Schiotz indents the cornea, aqueous is displaced.

53. b) The reading on the scale of a Schiotz tonometer must be looked up on a table and converted to mm mercury. FYI: The weights that come with each Schiotz tonometer are specific for that exact instrument, and are not interchangeable with another.

54. a) The eye of a young person or highly myopic person tends to be more elastic. This may result in a false low reading. (See questions 58-65.)

55. a) If the patient is squeezing, the eyelids can interfere with the interface between the instrument and the cornea. This causes a faulty reading. The IOP should be about the same regardless of which weight is used. See also question 82.

56. b) Each time the Schiotz is applied to the eye, a bit of aqueous is displaced (forced out). Repeated measurements could cause greater displacement and thus a falsely low reading.

57. a) High astigmatism can be a factor in applanation tonometry, not indentation. Repeating indentation measurements on a patient can force aqueous out of the eye, resulting in a falsely low reading. Squeezing the lids can interfere with the interface between the instrument and the cornea, causing a faulty reading. The eye of a young person or a highly myopic person tends to be more elastic, thus the eye would "give" during the measurement and give a falsely low reading.

58. a) Scleral rigidity refers to the elastic property (distensibility) of the sclera.

59. c) Something that is highly elastic would be less rigid. Of course, even a more distensible eye would still have some rigidity. Scleral rigidity affects the IOP *measurement*, not the IOP itself.

60. a) The displacement of aqueous that occurs during indentation tonometry causes distention of the eye's structures. The sclera of an eye with low rigidity (high elasticity) would "give", resulting in a falsely low reading.

61. b) See above.

62. c) Scleral rigidity in indentation tonometry can be identified by taking a reading with different weights, and comparing the results. (See question 63.)

63. a) If you've taken readings with different weights and find a difference of 3 mm Hg between them, suspect error due to scleral rigidity.

64. b) The applanation tonometer is not subject to scleral rigidity problems.

65. a) The applanation tonometer does not displace a significant enough amount of aqueous to cause even an elastic eye to distend.

66. c) Because the Schiotz comes in direct contact with the cornea and tear film, it must be cleaned between each patient.

67. a) Use a pipe cleaner dipped in alcohol or ether to clean the barrel of the Schiotz.

68. b) To sterilize means to kill all bacteria and spores. Alcohol and ether do not sterilize, but do disinfect.

69. b) Because the plunger touches the cornea and tear film, you would not want to contaminate it by touching it with bare fingers. Use gloves or a tissue.

70. d) Any chemical on the tonometer will be transferred to the cornea. A nasty chemical burn could result.

71. a) To kill bacteria and spores (sterilize), items *b* through *d* are adequate. An alcohol wipe will clean but not sterilize a surface. A 10-minute soak in 3% hydrogen peroxide is also acceptable.

72. d) The Schiotz tonometer is subject to erroneous readings when scleral rigidity is a factor. (See questions 58-65.) Otherwise, the Schiotz is not expensive and is easy to learn to use and calibrate.

73. c) Because it is small and portable, the Schiotz can be used at bedside. The other statements are false.

74. d) A test block is included with each instrument. To calibrate, hold the footplate against the test block at a 90 degree angle.

75. d) Some models have a nut screw that can be loosened to set the needle back to zero. Otherwise, the only way to have a Schiotz adjusted is to send it back to the manufacturer. Answers *a* through *c* may sound reasonable, but they don't work.

76. c) The patient must lie flat on his back for the reading.

77. c) Be careful not to press on the eye itself; this can cause a false reading. Use your fingers to gently pin the lids back toward the orbital rim.

78. c) With the Schiotz, the patient is lying back but the instrument position is still perpendicular to the central cornea.

79. b) The needle may pulsate slightly with the heartbeat (not breathing). Even with accurate alignment, there are other factors that can cause error, however.

80. d) Take the reading at mid-point between the measurements during the pulsations.

81. c) The Schiotz reading and IOP are inversely related, so a high Schiotz reading represents a low IOP.

82. c) If the reading is 2.5 or lower (remember, a low Schiotz reading indicates a high IOP), add more weight and repeat the measurement. (Be sure to use the proper chart then, when converting to mmHg.)

Chapter 7. Ocular Pharmacology

1. d) Anesthesia that puts the patient to sleep is known as general anesthesia. Topical anesthetic is applied to the skin (or eye), and local or regional is injected into a specific area.

2. b) Local anesthesia would be used in the chalazion excision. A baby cannot be relied upon not to move, so it needs to be totally asleep. Noncontact tonometry and topography are performed without any anesthetic.

3. a) In a regional block, anesthetic is injected into the area of the nerve (or nerves) that supplies the surgical site. An example would be a retrobulbar block, where the anesthetic is injected behind the eye to block sensation and to paralyze the muscles. Local anesthetic can also be injected into the tissues at the surgical site. "Site-specific local" is a bogus term.

4. b) A corneal transplant requires a regional block. The chalazion uses local, and topical is enough for radial keratotomy and laser trabeculoplasty.

5. b) Epinephrine causes blood vessels to constrict. This reduces bleeding at the surgical site. It also decreases systemic absorption of the drug, and keeps the anesthetic on location longer. Epinephrine has no effect on wound healing.

6. c) Hyaluronidase is used to increase the spread of the drug, causing a good, general coverage of the area. Unfortunately, this also means that systemic absorption is enhanced (a secondary, undesired side effect).

7. b) It often is necessary for the patient's eye to be immobilized, which can be accomplished with local anesthetic.

8. a) Lidocaine and procaine are commonly used local anesthetics. Answers *b* and *d* and tetracaine are *topical* anesthetics. Butane (in answer *c*) is used in cigarette lighters.

9. d) The most common side effect of local anesthetics is dizziness and nausea. Answers *a* and *b* can occur, but are not common. Blood pressure may be *reduced*, not increased; see next question.

10. a) Local anesthetics also may cause depression of both blood pressure and respiration.

11. c) The suffix "-caine" usually indicates that the drug is an anesthetic. Mannitol is an osmotic, cortisone is a steroid, and betaxolol is a beta blocker.

12. c) The initial contact lens fitting is not usually done with topical anesthetic. Lens fitters often use the patient's reaction to having lenses in the eye to help determine the patient's level of motivation.

13. a) The most common reaction to topical anesthetics is a contact allergic response. Some patients might experience dizziness and fainting, but this is not common. A decrease in blood pressure might occur on very rare occasions.

14. b) Proparacaine and tetracaine are the most commonly used topical anesthetics in ophthalmology. Drugs in answer *a* also are topical, but not used very often. Procaine, lidocaine, and prilocaine are local anesthetics, and epinephrine is sometimes an additive to local anesthetics.

15. d) The patient should be warned not to rub her eyes after the topical anesthetic has been instilled. Without corneal sensation, the patient might rub hard enough to cause a corneal abrasion.

16. b) Mydriatics are used to stimulate the dilator muscle of the iris and thereby cause pupil dilation. Mydriatics do not inhibit accommodation.

17. b) Because they dilate the pupil, mydriatics are used to facilitate fundus examination. Because they do not inhibit accommodation, they do not facilitate refractometry, although they might make retinoscopy (not given as an option) easier.

18. d) Phenylephrine is the most commonly used mydriatic. Tropicamide is a cycloplegic. Epinephrine and cocaine both have a mydriatic action (basically as a side effect), but are not used for dilation purposes.

19. a) Phenylephrine dilates the pupil in about 15 minutes and wears off in 1 to 2 hours. This makes it ideal for in-office use. (See Table 9-1.)

20. b) Phenylephrine is available in 2.5 and 10% concentrations. The weaker of the two, the 2.5% strength, is more commonly used and has fewer side effects than the 10% solution.

Table 9-1
Effect and Recovery of Dilation Drops

Diagnostic Drug	Time of Maximum Dilation	Time to Recovery
Phenylephrine	15 to 60 minutes	3 to 6 hours
Tropicamide/ hydroxyamphetamine	15 to 60 minutes	2 to 4 hours
Atropine	30 to 45 minutes	7 to 10 days
Homatropine	40 to 60 minutes	1 to 3 days
Scopolomine	20 to 30 minutes	3 to 7 days
Cyclopentalate	30 to 60 minutes	24 hours
Tropicamide	20 to 40 minutes	3 to 6 hours

Diagnostic Drug	Time of Maximum Cycloplegia	Time to Recovery
Atropine	30 to 50 minutes	5 to 12 days
Homatropine	30 to 70 minutes	1 to 3 days
Scopolomine	30 to 60 minutes	3 to 5 days
Cyclopentolate	30 to 45 minutes	24 hours
Tropicamide	60 to 180 minutes	6 hours

Reprinted with permission from Ledford JK, Pineda R. *The Little Eye Book: A Pupil's Guide to Understanding Ophthalmology.* Thorofare, NJ: SLACK Incorporated; 2002.

21. c) Diabetes, in the absence of other problems, is not a contraindication for mydriasis.

22. c) Cycloplegic agents paralyze both the ciliary muscle (thus inactivating accommodation) and the sphincter muscle of the iris (thus dilating the pupil).

23. c) Cycloplegics are used to facilitate retinoscopy and refractometry because of their accommodation deactivating ability. The fact that they dilate is almost secondary.

24. b) Cycloplegics are used in the treatment of iritis in order to halt painful accommodative spasms and to lessen the development of iris adhesions to the lens (posterior synechia).

25. See Table 9-1 for more details:
    A. The strongest drug   a
    B. Most rapid onset   e
    C. Wears off in 10 to 14 days   a
    D. Wears off in 1 to 3 days   b
    E. Wears off in 1 hour   e
    F. Used three times daily for 3 days before exam   a
    G. Wears off in 3 to 6 hours   d
    H. Weak; used more for dilation   e
    I. Duration falls between atropine and homatropine   c
    J. Onset 30 minutes   d

26. a) Systemic absorption of a cycloplegic may be accompanied by the symptoms of increased pulse, flushing, fever, and dry mouth (xerostomia).

27. b) Dark colored irises seem to be more resistant to cycloplegia, and thus may require more doses or stronger concentrations of the drug. (Use of a topical anesthetic prior to cycloplegic agents is a courtesy to any patient.)

28. b) A patient who is using a miotic, such as pilocarpine, will have a small pupil. The dilating/cyclo-plegic agent must counteract the miotic effect of the pilocarpine, so it may require more doses or stronger concentrations to achieve the desired effect. Propine is an epinephrine derivative, so if it has any effect on the pupil it would be to dilate it slightly. In general, beta blockers and CAIs do not have an effect on dilation.

29. c) All of the listed items are important; however, checking the patient's angles is the *most* important item of those listed. Admittedly, IOP should be taken before dilation, and perhaps after as well. Checking pupillary response is impossible after dilation. Refractometry might be required before and after cycloplegia. But dilating a patient with narrow angles could precipitate an angle-closure glaucoma attack.

30. b) Because accommodation and convergence are linked, any tests requiring binocular vision (eg, stereo testing, convergence, near point of accommodation) must be done prior to cycloplegia. While tonometry is ideally performed prior to any dilation, the measurement is not rendered *unreliable* by dilation.

31. a) Stinging and contact allergy are the most common side effects seen with use of mydriatics and cycloplegics. The other reactions might occur, but are not common.

32. b) Mydriatics and cycloplegics are packaged in bottles with red caps.

33. c) Epinephrine also is known as adrenaline. It is a chemical that occurs naturally in the body, and regulates the involuntary (sympathetic) nervous system. You might remember this as the "fight or flight" response. When threatened, adrenaline pours into the system, readying you for a confrontation or escape.

34. b) While topical epinephrine can cause pupil dilation, this is a secondary action. The primary use of topical epinephrine is in glaucoma treatment. Epinephrine is used in injectable (not topical) anesthetic to decrease wound bleeding. It is not used in treatment of dry eye.

35. c) Epinephrine derivatives used to treat glaucoma are preferred because they do not cause accommodative spasms and miosis, as do the miotics. Nor do they have as many systemic side effects as miotics. Miotics must be applied more often, a disadvantage. Epinephrine does not come in a gel as of this writing.

36. c) Iopidine is aproclonidine. The other drops listed are either epinephrine (Glaucon and Epinal) or contain epinephrine (P1E1 contains 1% pilocarpine and epinephrine).

37. c) Propine (generic name dipivefrin), is currently the most commonly used epinephrine derivative. Betagan and Timoptic are beta blockers, and Pilopine is pilocarpine in gel form.

38. a) Propine comes in 0.1%.

39. a) Side effects of epinephrine can include rapid pulse and respiration, stomach upset, pupil dilation, headache, fainting, increased blood pressure, and heart palpitations.

40. c) As indicated by the side effects listed in question 39, epinephrine is used with caution if the patient has cardiovascular disease, diabetes, or asthma.

41. b) Since a side effect of epinephrine can be pupil dilation, it should not be used in patients with narrow angles because an angle-closure glaucoma attack may occur.

42. b) Soperonol is contrived from my mother's maiden name. Answers *a, c,* and *d* are generic names for various beta blockers.

43. d) Iopidine is an alpha-2 agonist, not a beta blocker.

44. c) Beta blockers have blue or yellow caps.

45. c) The beta blockers classically have been contraindicated in patients with chronic obstructive pulmonary disease because the drugs can cause bronchospasms and decreased respiratory rate. The other statements are true. One or two beta blockers are approved for use once daily, but as a group they usually are given twice a day.

46. b) Because beta-blockers (even topical, ocular ones) can affect the heart, many physicians will require a baseline blood pressure and heart rate reading prior to beginning therapy, and on regular intervals thereafter.

47. d) Timoptic-XE is currently the only beta blocker gel that actually forms the gel when it is applied to the eye. Dosage is once daily, making it convenient.

48. a) Systemic beta blockers are used to treat congestive heart failure and hypertension. Examples are Tenormin, Lopressor, Toprol, and Inderal. They are not used for the other conditions listed, and are contraindicated in asthma.

49. c) Betoptic is a selective beta blocker, and less likely to have respiratory side effects.

50. a) Side effects of beta blockers (systemic or topical/ocular), as indicated above, can include decreased heart rate and decreased respiratory rate.

51. b) Other possible side effects of beta blockers include depression, insomnia, and impotence. Topical ocular beta blockers have minimal, if any, ocular side effects; over half of the people using them say they don't even sting. This contributes to their popularity.

52. c) Miotics stimulate the sphincter muscle of the iris, causing the pupil to close (miosis). This is suspected to pull on the trabecular meshwork (TM), but does not directly stimulate the TM. Stimulating the dilator muscle would cause dilation. Stimulating the ciliary body would cause increased aqueous production.

53. d) Miotics are not used in patients with posterior subcapsular cataracts because decreasing the pupil size would force the patient's visual axis straight through the cataract, drastically reducing vision. Miotics are used in open-angle glaucoma to lower IOP and in closed angle glaucoma to open the iris blockade. They are used in overcorrection (too much plus) following corneal refractive surgery. In addition, they reduce accommodative effort in convergent strabismus.

54. a) Miotics act to increase aqueous outflow.

55. d) Pilocarpine is the most often used miotic in IOP control.

56. c) Pilopine is 4% pilocarpine in a gel form. Timolol, while available as a gel (Timoptic XE) is a beta blocker, not a miotic.

57. c) Patients should be warned that they may experience a headache or brow ache when first starting a miotic. They should be encouraged to stick with treatment, as this side effect diminishes with use.

58. b) Miotics stimulate the sphincter muscle and "freeze" it in place; there are no spasms. Ciliary muscle spasms are the cause of the brow ache and headache experienced initially by some patients. Local allergic reaction can occur with any topical eye medication. Vision is decreased if cataracts are present because the smaller pupil forces the patient to try to look through the center of the lens, which often is the most dense part of the cataract (especially the posterior subcapsular type).

59. d) Systemic side effects of miotics include decreased blood pressure, cardiac arrest, sweating, and lethargy. Items in answer *b* are *local* side effects, not systemic side effects.

60. b) Dapiprazole is a miotic used in the office to reverse dilation.

61. a) The most common reactions to dapiprazole are stinging (over 50%) and redness (80%). The redness can last from 20 to 60 minutes.

62. c) Rev-Eyes (Bausch and Lomb) is the brand name of dapiprazole available at this printing. Paremyd is a little-used (and often unavailable) mydriatic. Phenoptic is a brand name of phenylephrine. Carabastat is the miotic carbachol.

63. c) Steroids are anti-inflammatory drugs, not anti-infectives. In fact, they can reduce the immune system and thus allow infections to occur. Steroids act to reduce swelling, redness, drainage, and scarring. They do not have an effect on bacteria or viruses. They can elevate the IOP and reduce immunity.

64. d) Herpes simplex is "fed" by steroids; thus, steroids in this case would make the infection worse. Steroids are used in Herpes zoster to treat resulting keratitis, conjunctivitis, and iritis. Iritis, scleritis, and episcleritis are all inflammatory conditions well treated by steroids.

65. d) Topical steroids usually are used for surface and anterior segment inflammation. Oral steroids are used for deeper ocular inflammations, such as posterior uveitis and optic neuritis. In some cases, scleritis might be treated with both topical and systemic steroids. Steroids can *cause* secondary glaucoma, so they are not used to treat it.

66. b) Diazepam is the generic term for Valium. All of the others are steroids. Betamethasone and cortisone acetate are two other steroids. (Often drug names ending in -one are steroids.)

67. a) Drugs in answer *b* are combination steroid-antibiotics. Answer *c* lists nonsteroidal anti-inflammatory drugs, and answer *d* is a list of antibiotics.

68. c) Steroids, whether topical or oral, are not discontinued suddenly. Instead, the dosage is tapered off gradually.

69. a) Because steroids can cause secondary glaucoma, the applanation tonometry test is the most important of those listed.

70. b) Steroids also can cause formation of posterior subcapsular cataracts. Hence the importance of the slit lamp exam.

71. d) Systemic side effects of steroids include sweating, elevated blood pressure, weakness, and delayed wound healing. They also can cause fluid retention, muscle wasting, bone demineralization, growth retardation, immunity suppression, and diabetes.

72. b) Steroids can lower the immune system, opening the tissues or system to opportunistic infection. They *can* increase blood glucose levels, and do *not* cause strokes.

73. a) Prolonged use of topical steroids (6 months or more) can cause the development of subcapsular cataracts. After 3 to 6 weeks of use, 8% of the population will experience a rise in their IOP. Other possible side effects include ptosis, mydriasis, and increased corneal thickness.

74. d) Steroids are often combined with antibiotics to fight both bacterial infection and inflammation. Examples are Poly Pred, Ak-Trol, and Maxitrol.

75. b) Antibiotics are used to treat bacterial infections.

76. b) Bacteriocidal antibiotics are those that actually kill bacteria. (Your hint of death is the suffix "-cidal.") Antibiotics that inhibit bacteria are called bacteriostatic, which includes the sulfonamides. An antiseptic inhibits germs and is used on surfaces.

77. c) See question 78. Penicillins are bacteriocidal. A germicide is used to kill bacteria on inanimate objects.

78. b) Penicillin, streptomycin, and ampicillin are bacteriocidal antibiotics. Drugs in answers *a* (antibiotics) and *c* (sulfonamides) are bacteriostatic. Drugs in answer *d* are antivirals, not antibiotics.

79. d) All of the brand names in answer *d* are sulfonamides, which are bacteriostatic. Brands in answer *a* are bacteriocidal, while those in answer *b* are antiviral. Answer *c* lists ocular lubricants.

80. c) One can determine the sensitivity of a germ to a particular antibiotic by taking a culture. Material from the infected tissue is spread on the culture plate. Tiny paper disks that have been impregnated with an antibiotic are spaced out on the plate. If the bacteria is sensitive to the antibiotic on a specific disk, there will be a zone of no growth around that disk. (A biopsy evaluates excised tissue. One cannot identify an antibiotic sensitivity by slit lamp or fluorescein angiogram.)

81. a) If an antibiotic has an effect on many different kinds of bacteria, it is called a broad spectrum drug. These are very useful when the infecting organism is not known, because chances are good that it will be sensitive to the drug.

82. d) An oral antibiotic should be taken until all the pills are gone.

83. c) The use of topical neomycin has been phased out (except in combination drugs) ecause of its high rate of allergic reaction.

84. c) Many people are allergic to sulfa drugs. AK-Sulf is a sulfonamide.

85. d) In general, antibiotics do not affect the blood glucose level. Any of the other answers are possible.

86. b) Up to 10% of the population is reportedly allergic to penicillin.

87. b) CAIs have the effect of lowering IOP.

88. d) CAIs act by reducing the amount of aqueous that is formed, thereby lowering IOP.

89. c) Acetazolamide is the generic name for Diamox. Mannitol is neither a brand name nor a CAI. Methazolamide and dichlorphenamide are no longer on the market.

90. a) Diamox is available as 500 mg sustained release sequels.

91. a) Lumigan is a prostaglandin. The rest are either a CAI (Trusopt and Azopt) or have a CAI in combination with another drug (CoSopt, which has timolol as well).

92. b) All of the items listed can occur as side effects of CAIs. However, tingling in the hands, feet, and tongue is so common that it has been suggested you can judge a patient's compliance by the presence (or absence) of this symptom.

93. b) Patients who are allergic to sulfa drugs should not take CAIs. Sulfa is an anti-infective. Sulfur is a chemical element, otherwise known as brimstone.

94. a) Vasoconstrictors cause constriction of blood vessels.

95. c) Vasoconstrictors make the conjunctival vessels smaller, thus whitening (getting the red out of) the eye. They do not have the effects listed in answers *a*, *b*, or *d*.

96. c) Another term for vasoconstrictors is decongestants.

97. b) Scopolamine is a cycloplegic agent. True, phenylephrine is a mydriatic drug, but it is also used in weaker concentrations as a decongestant.

98. a) Patients with dry eye should be discouraged from using vasoconstrictors, as these chemicals tend to dry the eye further. Hay fever and tired, red eyes can indicate the need for a decongestant. Using a decongestant in case of a subconjunctival hemorrhage won't really help the red to go away any faster, but is not contraindicated.

99. c) When an allergic reaction takes place, cells respond to the allergen by releasing histamine. Histamine is the chemical responsible for the redness, itching, watering, and rash seen in the typical allergic response. Antihistamines block the release of histamine. They cannot block the reaction, but do block some of the symptoms.

100. c) Opticrom is a mast call stabilizer.

101. b) Decongestants to reduce redness are frequently combined with antihistamines to alleviate allergy symptoms. Naphcon A and Vasocon-A are examples of such combinations.

102. c) Many oral antihistamines cause drowsiness. Many are available over the counter. Any drug can have systemic side effects. (In addition, a patient might be allergic to a preservative or other additive in such a medication.) Antihistamines are used to treat symptoms of allergies, not infections.

103. b) Oral and IV osmotics are used to lower the IOP rapidly in cases of angle-closure glaucoma. *Topical* osmotics are used in corneal edema. They are not indicated in open-angle glaucoma or tissue iritis.

104. a) If there is a permeable membrane separating two areas, then fluid will cross the system to equalize the fluid content on both sides of the membrane. If the membrane will allow fluids through but not particles, then the fluid will cross the membrane from the side with the least particles to the side with the most. Thus, the influx of fluid dilutes the particle concentration. This process is called *osmosis*. Osmotics raise the concentration of particles in the blood, which lowers the fluid content. Fluid (aqueous) then leaves the tissues (anterior chamber) and enters the blood stream in an attempt to equalize or dilute the concentration of particles.

105. d) Glycerin and isosorbide are sickly-sweet, and may cause nausea and vomiting if ingested quickly. Pour the liquid over ice and tell the patient to sip it slowly through a straw. If you dilute or follow the dose with water, you are adding water to the system and less fluid will be drawn out of the tissues.

106. a) Ismotic is a trade name for isosorbide. Isosorbide is not metabolized by the body as is glycerol. Therefore, it is safer to use in diabetic patients. Osmoglyn and Glyrol are brands of glycerol. Mannitol is an IV medication.

107. d) Mannitol and urea are the osmotics available for IV use. Glycerin and isosorbide are oral. Osmitrol is a trade name of mannitol, but glycerol is another name of the oral osmotic glycerin (so answer *b* is incorrect). Sucrose is sugar and lactose is milk sugar.

108. c) If a patient in angle-closure attack is being given oral osmotics and complains of thirst, she should be told that this means the medicine is working. The patient should not be given a drink, as this would reduce the amount of fluid being drawn out of the tissues. Giving more medication is done on doctor's orders only. Lying down won't help thirst.

109. b) Dehydration, headache, and disorientation are other side effects of systemic osmotics.

110. a) Topical osmotics act by creating high particle concentration (ie, low osmotic pressure) in the tears, which draws fluid out of the cornea.

111. c) Two or 5% sodium chloride (salt) drops or ointment (such as Muro 128) are frequently prescribed for home use in cases of long-term corneal edema.

112. b) In the office, a topical osmotic, such as anhydrous glycerin, can be applied to the eye to clear the cornea for examination. It has no appreciable effect on IOP.

113. a) Topical osmotics usually sting. They actually can clear vision temporarily (as long as the corneal edema is "dried up").

114. b) NSAIDs can offer relief of itching, but not other ocular allergic symptoms such as redness and watering. Items in answers *a*, *c*, and *d* are indications for topical NSAID use.

115. c) Prostaglandins are biochemicals that the body releases as a response to injury or other insult. The release of prostaglandins is responsible for the pain, fever, and swelling associated with the inflammatory response. NSAIDS act to reduce the formation of prostaglandins, thus reducing inflammatory symptoms.

116. a) NSAIDs do not appreciably elevate IOP, a significant problem in long-term use of steroids. The NSAIDs do not do a better job, are not combined with antibiotics, and do sting when instilled.

117. b) FML is a steroid eye drop. Answers *a*, *c*, and *d* are all topical NSAIDs.

118. b) NSAIDs are not indicated in an acute infection because in reducing the inflammation they may mask the advancement of the infection itself.

119. Matching:

Iopidine	f
Refresh	d
Tensilon	e
Healon	k
Polysporin	h
Lacrilube	d
Ocuvite	i
Viscoat	k
rose bengal	c
Viroptic	a
Gonak	j
Lacrisert	d
Tobradex	g
Ocuflox	h
fluorescein	c
Maxitrol	g
Quixin	h
Neosporin	h
Hypotears	d
Macugen	l
trypan blue	c
Goniosol	j
Ocucaps	i
acyclovir	a
Natacyn	b
Enlon	e

120. a) Fluorescein dye pools in corneal defects and glows in a cobalt blue light. You may use a blue filter on a pen light or on the slit lamp.

121. b) Rose bengal stains dead (necrotic) tissue, and would be of most use in a case of severe dry eye. It is of no use in glaucoma or conjunctival injection. Fluorescein dye would be more useful in the case of a corneal foreign body.

122. b) Vidarabine (Vira-A) seems to be effective only on the Herpes simplex virus.

123. d) The National Eye Institute's Age-Related Eye Disease Study (AREDS) shows that vitamins A, C, E, and zinc help slow down the progression of macular degeneration. (The NEI added copper and some antioxidants as well.) Hence the popularity of "eye vitamins" such as Ocuvite and ICaps.

124. b) Because there is no preservative to retard bacterial growth, any solution remaining in the bullet at the end of the day should be discarded. These drops may be used many times throughout the day. No one should use homemade saline in the eye because of the risk of contamination.

125. d) Dry eye is a condition that cannot be cured, only controlled. Thus, patients are advised to use the drops as often as needed.

126. a) Edrophonium chloride (Tensilon and Enlon) is used to diagnose myasthenia gravis. If the patient has myasthenia, an injection of Tensilon will cause the drooped lid to lift temporarily. It has no effect on congenital ptosis or levator weakness. Pilocarpine drops are used to identify Horner's syndrome.

127. c) Botulinum toxin (Botox) is used to relieve chronic lid twitching (blepharospasm). It also is used in some cases of nonaccommodative strabismus.

128. a) Prostaglandin analogues are substances that act like prostaglandins (which can either raise or lower IOP). In glaucoma treatment, prostaglandin analogues cause increased aqueous outflow. They seem to be more effective and have fewer side effects than beta-blockers. Currently marketed prostaglandin analogues are latanaprost (Xalatan), bimatoprost (Lumigan), and travoprost (Travatan).

129. b) Alpha-2 agonists are used to lower IOP. Examples are Iopidine and Alphagan.

130. b) The pH value is a way of talking about and measuring the acidity or alkalinity (base) properties of a substance. pH runs from 1 to 14, with less than 7 being an acid and over 7 a base (or alkaline). According to Duvall and Kershner,[2] a pH under 6.6 or over 7.8 causes discomfort when instilled into the eye. (By the way, the average pH of human tears is ~6.8.) *Buffers* are substances added to topical medications to alter the pH and bring it into a comfortable range.

131. a) *Buffers* are substances added to topical medications to control the pH range and salinity of the drug. *Preservatives*, which may be bacteriostatic (inhibit cell growth) or bacteriocidal (inhibit cell reproduction or kill cells), act to prevent bacterial contamination of medications. The *vehicle* is what "carries" the drug, that is an ointment (eg, white petrolatum), solution (eg, polyvinyl alcohol), a sterile paper strip (eg, fluorescein), etc. *Chelating agents* enhance the action of preservatives, making them more effective.

132. d) Another factor is expense of the drug. However, no medication perfectly fits each of these criteria. The physician will select the best one for each patient, often after a trial to find the most ideal.

133. b) Decreasing systemic absorption of topical eye medications is best done by reducing the amount of drug that enters the nasolacrimal system. The patient should close his eyes and gently press a finger into the medial nasolacrimal area for a minute or two. Any excess medication should be wiped away before opening the eyes.

Chapter 8. Photography

1. d) Every camera must include an aperture, camera body, and film. Believe it or not, a lens is not necessary, although it will make the resulting photograph much sharper.

2. d) While a camera does not have to have a lens, most do. The function of the lens is to focus the image onto the film. Some cameras incorporate minus (concave) lenses as part of the lens system, but their additive effect is convergent (a property of plus lenses).

3. a) In order to work at all, film must be sensitive to light. Grain size varies. The smaller the grain, the greater the detail of the images. The larger grain film is more sensitive to light. The "multipurpose" film used for snapshots is not suitable for medical and scientific photography.

4. c) Film speed is a measurement of the film's sensitivity. Film speed is rated by ISO numbers (previously ASA numbers); the higher the number, the faster and more sensitive the film. The more sensitive the film, the less exposure time is required. In addition, the faster film has larger silver grains in the film emulsion. This means that the slower films have better resolution, or detail.

5. b) See question 4.

6. a) See question 4.

7. b) Because the grain of a faster film is larger, there is poorer image quality.

8. b) Color slide film produces a positive image. In other words, the image of the object is imposed on the film exactly as it exists. The slides are created directly from the film; there are no negatives. In negative film, the prints are produced from negatives. This extra step causes a loss of resolution.

9. b) The size of the silver or dye particles in the film is known as grain. Finer grain produces sharper images. Larger grain reduces detail, and the photograph may even have a grainy appearance.

10. d) The contrast index of a film is a determination of the film's ability to produce variations of light and shadows. A high contrast film records mostly black and white; the photograph shows high contrast. Most of the real world is not high contrast, however, so a lower contrast index is more true to life.

11. b) The exposure of the film is a product of exposure length (how long light is allowed to hit the film, controlled by shutter speed) and the intensity of the light (controlled by aperture size, or f-stop, as well as available light or flashes). It does not have anything to do with film processing or the lens system.

12. d) In addition to the items mentioned in question 11, exposure is controlled by the sensitivity (speed) of the film and illumination intensity.

13. b) The f-stop controls the size of the diaphragm. The larger the f-stop, the larger the aperture, and the more light is allowed into the camera. Each higher f-stop setting increases the film exposure by a factor of two. Each lower shutter speed setting increases film exposure by a factor of two as well. (The settings represent fractions of a second. So 500 is 1/500 of a second; 250 is 1/250 of a second, which is half as fast.)

14. d) The shutter speeds are in fractions of a second, so a setting of 30 refers to 1/30 of a second.

15. b) There is no f-stop 0; 1 represents the aperture being wide open.

16. a) If the f-stop and shutter speed are not properly coordinated, the film may be overexposed or underexposed, but it *will* be exposed. It might not be worth processing, but it will be possible to process it.

17. c) The focal length of a camera lens is the distance from the lens to the film plane. As in optics, this represents the distance from the lens to the focal point. In this case, the focal point falls on the film.

18. a) A telephoto lens has a longer focal length. This has the effect of bringing distant objects closer by magnifying them. A normal lens gives a 1:1 ratio (ie, images appear life-sized). A wide-angle (micro) lens has a short focal length, and is used to give a wider field.

19. c) The zoom lens is adjustable, and thus has varying focal lengths. The Soper lens is a type of contact lens for keratoconus. The macro and micro lenses are not adjustable, having a fixed focal length.

20. c) Depth of field refers to the area in which objects are in acceptable focus.

21. d) One-third of the depth of field is usually in front of the focused subject (point of focus) and two-thirds are behind. Thus, if the depth of focus is 3 ft, objects that are within 1 ft in front of the subject will still be focused, and objects that are within 2 ft behind the subject still will be focused.

22. b) The depth of field can be extended by using a larger f-stop. By contrast, a smaller f-stop will decrease the depth of field. (Remember, this deals with objects in front of or behind the subject, not to the sides.)

23. a) As long as the f-stop is kept constant, depth of field also can be manipulated by using a wide-angle lens, which has a short focal length. A standard 50 mm lens has a longer focal length, and a telephoto lens has a longer focal length yet.

24. c) The shorter the camera to subject distance, the shallower the depth of field.

25. c) Shutter speed does not affect depth of field.

26. b) Synchronization refers to the flash emitting its brightest at the same time that the shutter is maximally open.

27. a) If synchronization is off, only part or none of the film may be exposed. The shutter will close before the light is brightest, or the shutter doesn't open until after the light is brightest.

28. b) An electronic flash should be connected to the X outlet on the camera. The M outlet is for flashbulbs. The FP is used for flashbulbs with a focal plane shutter. There is no KH outlet.

29. a) The beam splitter uses prisms to split the image into two: one for the oculars and one for the camera.

30. d) See question 29.

31. b) Because the beam splitter diverts some of the light, the amount of light that comes through the oculars is reduced. This also reduces detail. In cameras where the beam splitter can be flipped out of the way, it must be flipped back into place *before* the photograph can be taken.

32. a) In fundus cameras, the image that the photographer views is focused in space. The reticule is needed to give a reference point for focusing. The reticule and subject must be in focus simultaneously. The ocular is set for the photographer's refractive error, not necessarily at zero. Unless the patient is a high myope (or external pictures are being taken with the fundus camera), the dioptric setting should be plano. FYI: *Reticule* and *reticle* are the same thing: a grid or ruler inscribed in the ocular (eyepiece) of a camera or other piece of optical equipment for focusing and measuring. It is not printed on the photograph.

33. c) The reticule is designed to be focused at infinity. This relaxes the photographer's accommodation.

34. d) See question 32.

35. b) The eyepiece should be set in dim light (or in the dark) with both eyes open. On the fundus camera, this means that one eye is looking through the eyepiece and the other eye is not. This is difficult to do, perhaps, but best.

36. b) The fundus camera ocular is set like any other eyepiece. Turn it all the way to plus. Looking through the eyepiece, turn slowly toward the minus. Stop when the image is clear. Do not pass the clear spot in search of more clarity. It is not necessary to remove your correction. But if you wear your glasses sometimes, and other times don't, you'll have to reset the ocular.

37. c) Going past the first point of image clarity adds minus to the ocular, which forces your eye to add plus (accommodate) to compensate. The resulting photographs will not be clear. You are not compensating for the patient's refractive error, but your own.

38. c) The patient's optical media become part of the camera's lens system. If there is a corneal or lenticular opacity, the photographs will not be clear. The dioptric power of the eye cannot be discounted. If the patient is a high myope or hyperope, the dioptric compensation device must be set. Some fundus cameras have a compensation device for astigmatism, as well.

39. a) An image that seems to vary in focus probably is due to the accommodation of the photographer. Have the patient sit back, and check the focus of your ocular(s) again.

40. a) A blue-gray halo around the subject indicates that you are too far back. Move the camera closer. If you are too close, you will see a whitish haze in the center of the subject.

41. d) See question 40. The whitish central haze means you are too close.

42. b) Gross focusing can be accomplished by moving the joy stick. On some fundus cameras, fine focusing is accomplished by turning a focusing knob on the camera. The subject is never focused by turning the oculars or by asking the patient to move. Changing the magnification setting will make the image larger, but not more focused.

43. c) If the fundus camera donut is focused on the patient's closed lid, you are going to be very close to being in focus when the patient opens her eye. Moving the camera around to search for the subject is not very professional or practical, nor very comfortable for the patient who must endure the bright light that much longer. If the fixation light is in front of the camera, it will get in the way of the photograph.

44. b) Video recordings are great because they provide instant play-back. However, the resolution (sharpness) of the images isn't great, especially when a frame is paused. Compared to other pieces of ophthalmic equipment, video equipment is inexpensive and uncomplicated. Videotapes are copied easily, but resolution is lost with copying.

45. b) There is no need to use videotaping for pachymetry.

46. c) In some shots needed for fundus photography (notably during diabetic fields, or to document peripheral lesions), the angle of incidence between the camera and cornea can induce astigmatism. This can cause blurring of the photograph in one meridian. Accommodation is spherical, not cylindrical.

47. c) See question 46.

48. a) Some fundus cameras have an astigmatic correction device that is used much like the dioptric compensation setting. The dioptric compensation device is spherical refractive errors, not cylindrical. The difficulty of fitting a toric contact lens just for photography makes it a poor option.

49. c) Check the eyepiece! (That is the first rule when using any piece of focusable eye equipment.) If the lens isn't dirty, don't touch it. Homatropine is not necessary for dilation; usually, weaker drops are used. The dioptric compensator should be set on a patient-by-patient basis.

50. c) Four to 5 mm dilation would be the minimum size for fundus photos. (8 mm would be best, of course, but it is not the *minimum*.)

51. d) It is important to continue to encourage the patient throughout the entire photography session.

52. d) To scan the patient's retina, swing the camera on its pivot. If you move the joystick, you are moving the camera base. If the patient follows the fixation light or moves his chin, you are going to lose your field of view.

53. a) The primary component of the optical imaging system of the fundus camera is an aspheric lens that acts as an indirect ophthalmoscope. (A retinoscope is used in refractometry, remember?)

54. c) The view lamp and the electronic flash system make up the illumination exposure system. A beam splitter is part of a slit lamp camera system. Only tungsten bulbs are used. The fixation light does not play a role in exposing the film.

55. c) If the patient is highly hyperopic or myopic beyond the normal focusing ability of the camera, the diopter compensation device is used.

56. d) A visual field test is not a prerequisite for having fundus photos.

57. b) If you set the dioptric compensation device to "+" it is possible to take a photo of the external eye using the fundus camera.

58. b) Have the patient close both eyes while you align the donut on the closed lid. This is more comfortable for the patient and allows you to avoid fumbling around with the camera looking for the eye.

59. a) The orange-yellow background color of the fundus should be even across the viewing field.

60. b) Ask the patient to blink just before you fire the camera. This clears the tear film and increases the chances of the lids being open widely when you snap the picture.

61. b) Fundus photography is used in all of the listed situations except aphakia. Aphakia is a condition, not a disease, and does not require photographic monitoring.

62. a) The optic disc is the primary object of interest in monitoring glaucoma patients.

63. c) The diabetic survey includes pictures of seven overlapping fields.

64. c) Allow the patient to rest briefly between photos of both eyes. This allows her to recover from being "dazzled" before being required to see the fixation light.

65. d) The little yellow crescent is caused by a "pupil cut."

66. b) To compensate for a pupil cut, move the camera directly opposite from the crescent.

67. c) Retinal pathology does not cause blurred photos in and of itself.

68. b) In addition to causing pupil cuts, inadequate dilation can cause a general blur on the photographs.

69. Matching:
    A. Camera too close   f, Figure 8-6
    B. Camera too far back   c, Figure 8-3
    C. Film not completely advanced   a, Figure 8-1
    D. Flash not synchronized with shutter   d, Figure 8-4
    E. Patient blinked   e, Figure 8-5
    F. Pupil cut   b, Figure 8-2

252 Chapter 9

References

1. Gordon MO, Beiser JA, Brandt JD, et al. The ocular hypertension treatment study: baseline factors that predict the onset of primary open-angle glaucoma. *Arch Ophthalmol.* 2002;120:714-720.
2. Duvall B, Kershner R. *Ophthalmic Medications and Pharmacology.* Thorofare, NJ: SLACK Incorporated; 1998. pg. 2.

Answers by Category and Suggested Readings

This section is included so that the prospective ophthalmic technician can identify weak areas. In addition, those interested in taking the exams for Certified Paraoptometric (CPO), Certified Paraoptometric Assistant (CPOA), Certified Paraoptometric Technician (CPOT), American Board of Opticianry Certification (ABOC), National Contact Lens Examination (NCLE), Certified Retinal Angiographer (CRA), and ophthalmic surgical assisting subspecialty (Srg), can identify those section that apply to them. There are advanced levels for NCLE and ABOC, but the candidate would have already mastered the knowledge and tasks at this (COT®) level.

Chapter 2. Clinical Optics

1-52. Optics
    CPOA: Optical Crosses, Optics
    CPOT: Optical Principles of Light, Optical Crosses
    ABOC: Basic level
53-82. Retinoscopy
83-134. Refractometry
135-170. Advanced Spectacle Principles
    CPOA: Vertex Distance, Prism, Aphakic
    CPOT: Prism, Vertex Distance, Aphakia
    ABOC: Basic level
171-183. Low Vision Aids
    CPOT: Low Vision

Chapter 3. Basic Ocular Motility

1-11. Extraocular Muscle Actions
    CPOA: Eye Movements (Definitions)
    CPOT: Eye Movements
12-46. Strabismus
    CPOT: Binocular Vision (Disorders)
47-53. Amblyopia Detection
    CPOT: Refractive Conditions (Amblyopia)
54-166. Evaluation Assessment Methods
    CPOA: NPC, Fusion, Stereo Acuity
    CPOT: Muscle Balance, NPC, Fusion, Stereo Acuity

Chapter 4. Visual Fields

1-22. Visual Pathways
    CPOA: Visual Pathway
    CPOT: Visual Pathway
21-40. Visual Fields (definitions)
    CPOT: Terminology
41-50. Methods (Screening and Threshold)
51-181. Techniques (Manual, Kinetic, Static, Automated)
    CPOA: Visual Fields
    CPOT: Visual Fields (Instrumentation)

182-187. Errors
188-222. Visual Field Defects
      CPOT: Classification of Defects

Chapter 5. Contact Lenses

The category in general:
      NCLE: Basic level
1-102. Basic Principles
      CPO: Soft, Rigid
      CPOA: Terminology, Special Lens Designs
      CPOT: Types, Special Lens Design
103-156. Fitting Procedures
      CPOT: Keratometry, Pre-Fitting Evaluation, Fitting Theories
157-192. Patient Instruction
      CPO: Care and Handling, Patient Education
      CPOA: Care and Handling
      CPOT: Care and Handling Techniques
193-250. Trouble Shooting Problems
      CPOA: Solutions
      CPOT: Solutions, Modification, Related Ocular Problems
251-270. Verification of Lenses
      CPO: Parameters, etc.
      CPOA: Verification
      CPOT: Verification

Chapter 6. Intermediate Tonometry

1-7. Aqueous Humor Dynamics
8-50. Glaucoma
      CPOA: Disorders (Glaucoma)
      CPOT: Eye (Pathology/Glaucoma)
      Srg: Surgical Procedures (Glaucoma Surgery, Laser Surgery)
51-82. Indentation Tonometry
      CPOA: Tonometry (Indentation)
      CPOT: Tonometry (Indentation)

Chapter 7. Ocular Pharmacology

The category in general:
      COPT: Pharmacology
      CRA: Ocular Pharmacology
1-15. Anesthetics
      CPOA: Anesthetics
      Srg: Ophthalmic Anesthesia
16-32. Mydriatics and Cycloplegics
      CPOA: Mydriatics, Cycloplegics
      Srg: Mydriatics

33-41. Epinephrine
42-51. Beta-Blockers
52-62. Miotics
    CPOA: Miotics
    Srg: Miotics
63-74. Steroids
75-86. Antibiotics
87-93. Carbonic Anhydrase Inhibitors
94-98. Vasoconstrictors
99-102. Antihistamines
103-113. Osmotic Agents
    Srg: Osmotic Diuretics
114-118. Nonsteroidal Anti-inflammatories
119-133. Others (*Note*: We have included diagnostic stains, antivirals, prostaglandin analogues, etc.).
    CPOA: Stains
    Srg: Viscoelastics, Other

Chapter 8. Photography

The category in general:
    CPOT: Ocular Photography
    CRA: General Photography, Fundus Photography
1-48. Basics of Photography
49-64. Fundus Photography
65-69. Defects/Artifacts

Suggested Readings

Cassin, B, ed. *Fundamentals for Ophthalmic Technical Personnel.* Philadelphia, Pa: Saunders; 1995.

Choplin N, Edwards, R. *Visual Fields.* Thorofare, NJ: SLACK Incorporated; 1998.

Cunningham D. *Clinical Ocular Photography.* Thorofare, NJ: SLACK Incorporated; 1998.

Duvall B, Kershner RM. *Ophthalmic Medications and Pharmacology.* Thorofare, NJ: SLACK Incorporated; 1998.

Gayton JL, Ledford JR. *The Crystal Clear Guide to Sight for Life.* Lancaster, Pa: Starburst; 1996.

Hansen VC. *A Systematic Approach to Strabismus.* Thorofare, NJ: SLACK Incorporated; 1998.

Ledford JK. *Handbook of Clinical Ophthalmology for Eyecare Professionals.* Thorofare, NJ: SLACK Incorporated; 2001.

Lens A. *Optics, Retinoscopy, and Refractometry.* Thorofare, NJ: SLACK Incorporated; 1999.

Riordan-Eva P, Whitcher JP, eds. *Vaughn & Asbury's General Ophthalmology.* 16th ed. New York, NY: Lange Medical Books/McGraw-Hill; 2004.

Stein HA, Slatt BJ, Stein RM. *The Ophthalmic Assistant: A Guide for Ophthalmic Medical Personnel.* 7th ed. San Diego, CA: Harcourt Publishers; 2000.

Printed in the United States
by Baker & Taylor Publisher Services